Woven into the fabric

of a broken heart

are stories of great love

and deep sorrow.

The Art of
GRIEVING

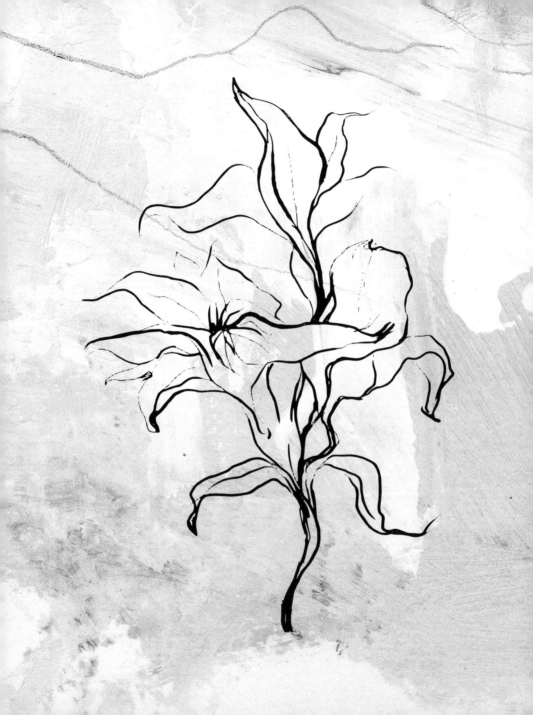

The Art of
GRIEVING

CORINNE LAAN

GENTLE SELF-CARE PRACTICES
TO HEAL A BROKEN HEART

ROCKPOOL

A Rockpool book
PO Box 252
Summer Hill
NSW 2130
Australia

rockpoolpublishing.com

Follow us! **f** 🄾 rockpoolpublishing
Tag your images with #rockpoolpublishing

ISBN: 9781922579201

Published in 2022 by Rockpool Publishing

Design by Daniel Poole, Rockpool Publishing
Illustrations by Natalya Tugova
Edited by Lisa Macken

A catalogue record for this
book is available from the
National Library of Australia

Printed and bound in China
10 9 8 7 6 5 4 3 2 1

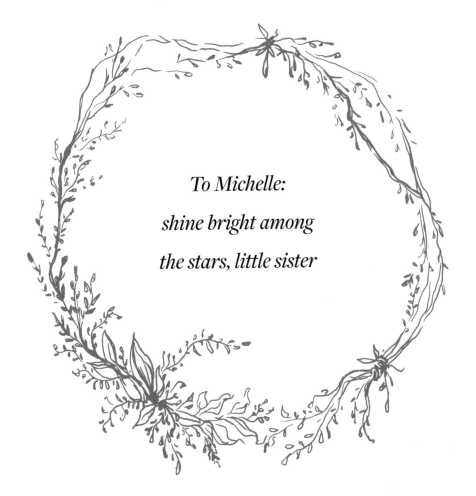

To Michelle:

shine bright among

the stars, little sister

The world you once knew changed in a second

That is all it took to knock the breath out of you

There is no safe place to lay your

wounded soul to rest

There is no fight left in you

Your heart shatters in silent little pieces

No one hears your cries

No one wants to listen to your anguish

You are alone

Push down your emotions into the abyss

where your heart once resided

Make your grief invisible to the outside world

Until a new day appears on the horizon

And you feel the comforting

touch of the sun again

Feel the fresh breeze of something

fleetingly different

A new tide has arrived

The promise of light after darkness is here

Lift your gaze towards the stars

And explore the mystery the universe holds

Bring along your wounded heart

Take a deep breath

Slow down

And

Grieve.

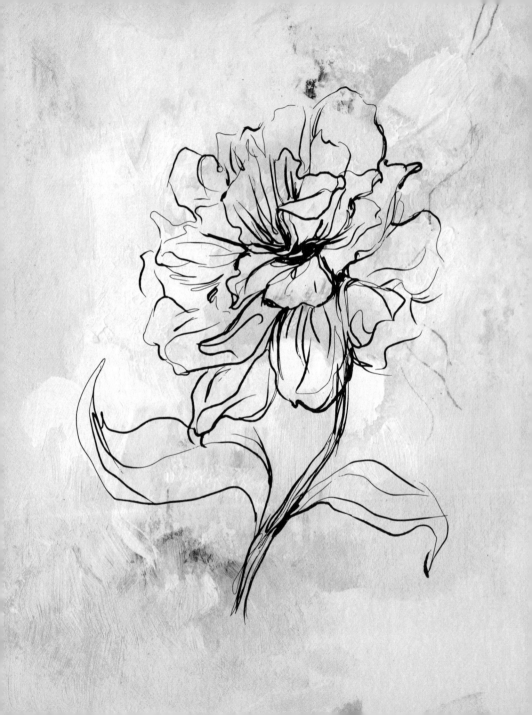

Preface
a note on death

A place to stay untouched by Death does not exist.
It does not exist in Space, it does not exist in the Ocean.
Nor if you stay in the middle of a mountain.

– Gautama Buddha

This book includes self-care practices that can be used for all types of grief; however, I would like to add a special note about death because I sense there is a real need to open up the conversations surrounding death. Especially this past year, during which we were struck by a global pandemic and could not be there in person for those we love. Most importantly, we are grieving alone.

We live in a society that has great difficulty talking about death, and over the years we have lost our connection to death. Nowadays there are few rituals concerning death and burial ceremonies are quickly dealt with. We are expected to get over any loss swiftly and move on because we feel that expressing our grief is a sign of weakness and overt mourning is too awkward for onlookers to witness. These aspects of mourning have crept into our perception of what is regarded as normal around death because the rituals and ceremonies around it have disappeared over the years. Death has become unfamiliar despite it occurring every minute of the day.

Facing death means we have to recognise our own mortality, that we have to admit our time in this world is limited. We have to accept the fact that life is fragile and a gift that is denied to many.

In some unfortunate ways we have lost our ability to truly be present in our own grief and be of support to the griever. As death continues to be pushed into the shadows, finding a shoulder to lean on while grieving is becoming more and more challenging.

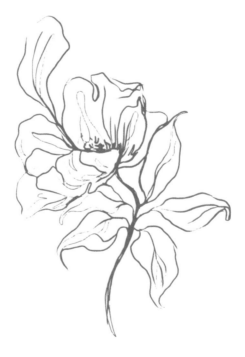

We have to accept

the fact that life is

fragile and a gift that

is denied to many.

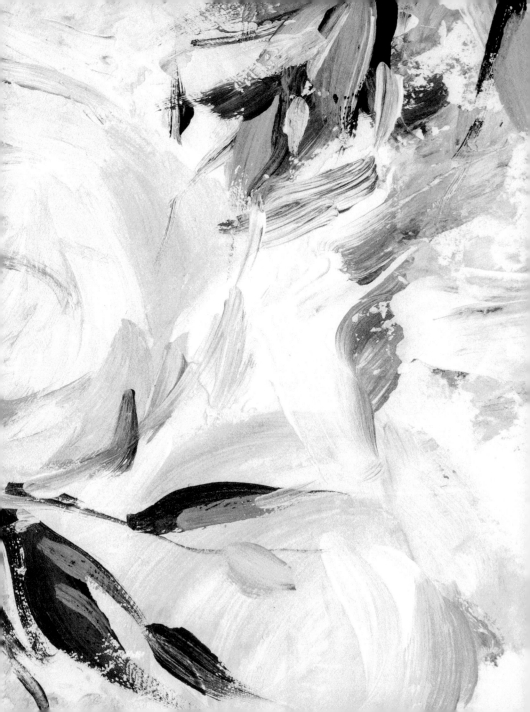

Contents

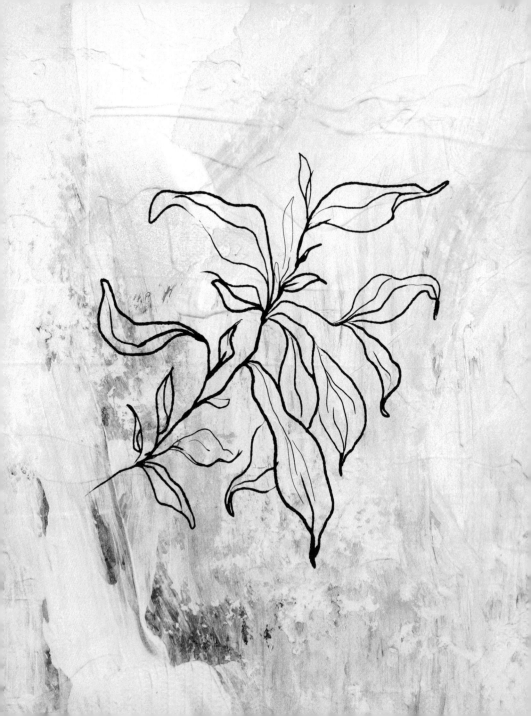

I

My story
the beginning

I first captured a vision of this book during an early morning walk along a sandy beach many years ago. The vision flash was as quick as lightning, but just before it disappeared it left an imprint as clear as day: it would be a book about healing.

The mystery of the book was intriguing and had me thinking hard about it on my way home. Although I did not consider myself a writer I made summaries of my thoughts in my notebook. I had never written anything of substance before and the thought of writing a book did at first seem daunting. I didn't know what to make of my vision but one thing I remembered clearly was that there is a lot of healing to be done. Whether my thoughts indeed became a book or part of the work I do, I knew I needed to get started right away and then the how and when would unfold. I had to trust the path ahead.

The book took shape over the years amid life-changing experiences. For instance, my then five-year-old son contracted a serious lung infection that nearly took his life. The days and nights spent at the hospital watching his little body fight the infection were a frightening reminder of how fragile life is. My own health experienced a nose dive when what should have been day surgery took a turn for the worse and I ended up spending a few days in hospital. My surgeon said I had been lucky, and her colleague later told me that if it had not been for my surgeon's skilled hands I would have ended up in intensive care. That same year my father, the strongest man I ever knew, died after a short illness. The cancer proved too powerful and his body did not respond to treatment. Watching him fade away until he became a man I did not recognise left me feeling helpless and angry.

It was a year of turmoil and grief. How unfair life can be at times! As life began to find its balance and flow I developed my own way of working with grief and healing. At the beginning I shared some of my written work with mothers who were grieving and I found that the more I shared the more I became encouraged to write and let my creativity loose. Elizabeth Gilbert's book *Big Magic* was a source of great inspiration in my early stages of sharing my writing with the world. Looking back, I believe there was a process I had to go through that meant leaving the fear of rejection behind so my original vision could take physical shape in the form of an actual book.

I feel this book has always been with me, from back in the 1970s and well before my fateful walk on the beach watching the sun come up over the horizon. A few weeks short of my seventh birthday my sister Michelle, who was only four days old, died. She was perfect; she was my beautiful baby sister. We had just welcomed her and the excitement of having a brand new baby, a new family member, was thick in the air. There was so much joy the day she was born, and then just like that she was gone. The pain of losing her lives on and never truly goes away. Memories of her are forever imprinted in my heart and mind and sadly are all I have left of her. Some days I can close my eyes and see her clearly while on other days the images are blurry, and on those days I panic in fear I will forget what she looked like.

What remains without a shadow of a doubt is the seven-year-old me: deeply wounded and trying desperately to make sense of what happened. One minute my father and I were picking up my baby sister and mother from hospital – I remember sitting in the back of the car, my gaze never once leaving my sister and my father happily chatting away with his friend – then, out of the blue, Michelle was gone. We buried her in a tiny white coffin. It did not make sense to me: why her, why us? The 'why' haunted me for a long time, and I recall being unable to talk to my mother about Michelle's death because it made her cry and I would blame myself. The only person I could talk to at the time was my father.

This very early experience of infant death shaped my path and my career choice. I chose to become a nurse, and I gravitated towards working with mothers and babies very early in my career.

In my current work as a practitioner of traditional Chinese medicine I support women as they seek to work through all types of grief, which is very often the cause of many of the physical ailments my clients face. I see women who are grieving the loss of a loved one, are experiencing fertility issues, are going through the hardship of a divorce or have lost a whole community when they settled in a foreign country. During the current pandemic I felt a collective grief gathering force due to physical distancing and the fact we mostly had to grieve alone, all of which adds to the emotional trauma we carry. Business owners lost their livelihoods, people lost jobs and contracts, each and every one of us lost our freedom and the lives we were used to. In the end, we are all grieving the loss of something that was once precious to us.

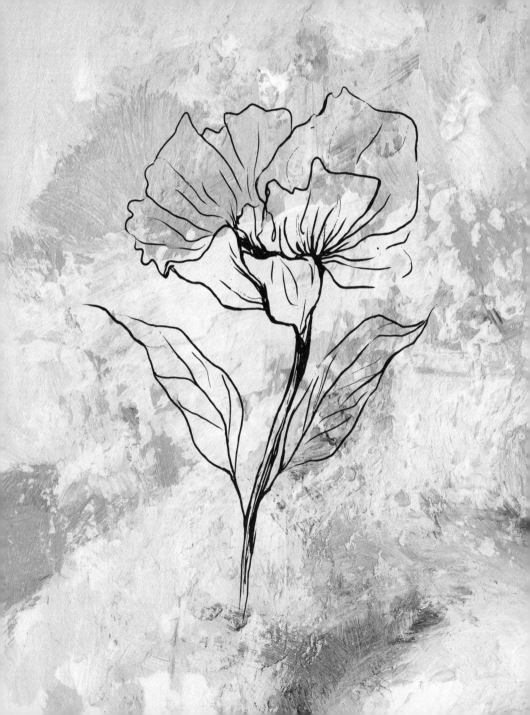

II

How to use this book

a gentle guide on your healing journey

You may have chosen this book because you were attracted by the cover and title, you felt called to it or you were intrigued by what might be written inside. Whatever the reason, I would like to give you a warm welcome. You are ready to embrace your grief and heal your broken heart. Many readers will be able to process their grief on their own, but if the pain and emotions you are experiencing are too overwhelming please do seek help from a grief counsellor who can help you on your journey. I offer within some healing self-care practices, which I refer to as rituals, for you to explore, and you can use these rituals to help you further on your grieving and healing journey.

Some of the rituals can be undertaken at home, while others are outdoor rituals. If you are new to rituals and find the idea of performing them outdoors daunting, start with the ones you can easily do at home. Once you have built your confidence you can incorporate the outdoor rituals.

This book is not meant to be read from cover to cover but rather to be used as a gentle guide on your healing journey. My advice is to choose a ritual that engages your curiosity and resonates with you on a deeper level.

I have included a special section for women who are facing fertility issues, and the silent grief that comes with this journey, and for mothers who have experienced pregnancy loss, a subject that is close to my heart.

Skip any pages that feel less relevant to you and go to the ones you need in the moment. Feel free to elaborate and add your uniqueness to the rituals; in fact, I encourage you to do so. You can create your very own ritual that holds special meaning for you. As you turn the pages I wholeheartedly invite you to dive deeper into the magic of rituals.

I hope the gentle practice of self-care rituals gives your sorrow the space it needs to create the transformation you are seeking. It is only through embracing and expressing your grief that you can eventually begin to heal the fragmented pieces of your heart and start to feel whole again. My biggest hope is that you will find solace, inspiration and comfort within the pages of this book. May you feel my comforting presence as I accompany you through each and every page.

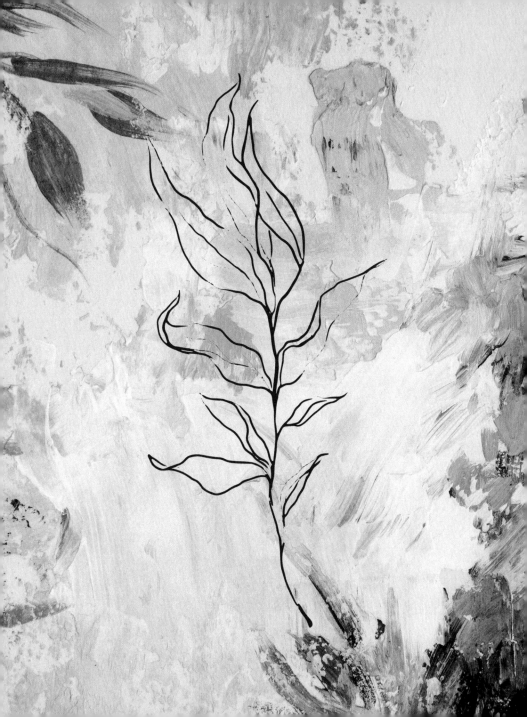

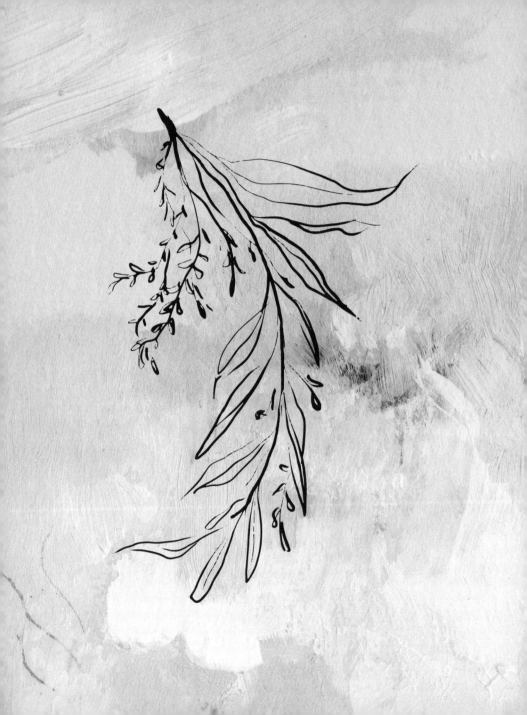

1

What is grief?

when love meets loss

It is difficult to talk about grief and the myriad of emotions that arises following a loss. It is a territory many feel ill-equipped to handle for fear of saying or doing the wrong thing, which can leave the person grieving feeling as though they have been abandoned. We live in a society that values strength, which means that any show of emotion is viewed as being an act of weakness. Grief and mourning have to be dealt with swiftly then neatly filed away somewhere so we can go back to 'normal' as soon as possible – whatever we perceive normal to be. The fast-paced lives we lead make incredible demands on us at the detriment of our healing and long-term well-being. There is no time or place for sorrow; we must pursue joy and happiness at all cost.

A broken heart deserves better than a quick fix. We are not machines that can be mended by replacing a malfunctioning part; we are souls living in human form, we are living, breathing, emotional beings. Regardless of the pressure placed upon us by our community, society or culture we must slow down and fully attend to our fragmented hearts. We must create the space to grieve and mourn in order for deep healing to take place. This means restoring to a state of well-being both our bodies and minds as well as our souls. To find deep peace within chaos we need to stop and take the time to attend to all of the emotions that arise, including the ups and the downs that follow a loss. We need to pay attention and be aware of our body's needs and take good care of our mental and spiritual well-being, not only for our own sakes but for the sakes of those who depend on us.

We often think of grief as merely an emotional response to loss; however, it has many different layers. Grief affects us physically, mentally and spiritually, and has social, cultural and even philosophical and psychological implications that unfortunately are very often overlooked or cast aside. Grief affects individuals on many, many levels and we are often bewildered about how to deal with our own grief, let alone someone else's.

Grief is as unique to an individual as are their fingerprints. It is a natural process that is the result of loving deeply. We grieve because love is our blueprint. Although we often share similarities with other people, grief remains a unique and personal journey. It can be a lifelong process, and there is no right or wrong way to mourn a loss. There is no quick-fix magic formula to end grief: it becomes part of you, but there are ways in which you can live a good life while still grieving.

Although grief is a normal process, it is important to recognise the negative impact it can have on your health and relationships if it is not properly addressed. Grief cannot be put aside and dealt with later, because while it is shut away it brews and gathers incredible momentum and can strike with the force of a powerful storm when you least expect it.

We often hear the phrase 'time heals all wounds', but from what I have witnessed while working with grief this is not true. Time does *not* heal grief. Instead, time offers us the space to mourn, to reflect and to explore ways to deal with the sorrow. Time actually transforms grief into something a broken heart can bear, providing us the space to gradually move towards new adjustments, hope, acceptance and healing.

Grief changes who we are, which is the scariest thing about it. Not only do we have to learn to live with the pain, but we are no longer the person we used to be and cannot ever go back to being that person. Everything has changed and we are forever changed. It is critical that we learn to live with grief and the loss of the person we used to be.

The complications of grief

There are so many different types of grief we may experience, and they will not always be associated with the loss of a loved one but can also apply to different areas of our lives whereby we lost something we held close to our hearts. It is beyond the scope of this book to explore in detail all of the varying types of grief; however, below is a short explanation of some types that can affect us.

- **Normal grief** usually lasts between six months to a year.
- **Prolonged grief** occurs when intense sorrow extends beyond 12 months and starts to affect physical and mental health.
- **Anticipatory grief** occurs when a loved one is expected to die as the result of an illness or following an accident, for example. Anxiety and fear often accompany this type of grief as the future may seem uncertain and you have to imagine living your life without this person. Anticipatory grief can also be related to a job contract or close friendship coming to an end.

- **Cumulative or compounded grief** is grief that piles up due to recurrent losses, deaths and traumatic life events.

- **Collective grief** is felt by a whole community, city, country or world, for example, the COVID-19 pandemic. Other examples include war, natural disasters and the death of an important public figure.

- **Disenfranchised grief**, which I refer to as 'invisible grief', is not recognised by society and therefore support is hard to find. It is often felt by women who are experiencing fertility issues, have suffered a miscarriage or had an abortion, or have an illness that has resulted in a deterioration of physical fitness.

- **Delayed grief** takes a while to manifest because you need to be strong for your own survival or have to take care of other people around you. This type of grief is experienced after a divorce or the loss of a job as well as following the death of a loved one.

- **Distorted grief** occurs when you experience intense or extreme emotion that manifests in self-destructive behaviour or hostility towards others.

- **Exaggerated grief** intensifies over a period a time and can result in mental health disorders that affect several areas of your life. Some of the symptoms that may increase include nightmares, suicidal thoughts, phobias and self-destructive behaviour.

- **Traumatic grief** follows the abrupt loss of a loved one through a horrific accident or violent event. The distress caused by this type of grief can impair daily life.

- **Masked grief** occurs when the griever keeps their grief hidden from the outside world.

- **Inhibited grief** occurs when you exhibit just a few signs of grief but hold most of your pain internally. This triggers the grief to instead reveal itself in physical form via symptoms such as headaches, nausea and general aches and pains.

- **Abbreviated or shortened grief** occurs when the griever seems to have moved on very quickly from the initial loss. This is often seen in cases of divorce or the death of a loved one.

- **Absent grief** occurs when the bereaved does not show any signs of grieving. Initially, this can be normal due to the suddenness of the loss and before reality has set in, but over time it can become concerning.

It is important to identify the type of grief you are experiencing and seek the guidance of a health professional to help you process it. You can use the gentle self-care practices in this book as an additional tool to make the changes you desire to restore your emotional and physical health.

Healing after loss

Healing may mean different things to different people and may also look different, but it has one common theme: getting better.

Healing may seem simple, yet it is a complex process that often involves many intricate aspects and phases coming together in perfect synchronicity. In straightforward terms healing means finding relief and getting and feeling better, which can be felt physically, emotionally and spiritually.

Healing is not an easy process and nobody knows how long it will take for any individual to start feeling better. However, one thing is for sure: healing needs your active participation, and possibly even your complete devotion. It can be hard work and it requires intention, focus, support, faith, understanding, compassion, empathy and a large dose of love. Healing from any type of loss is a lifelong commitment. Although the work of healing yourself is always ongoing, it can be seen as a promise to be restored, a pledge to feel joy again. I hope the self-care practices outlined in this book will help you become an active participant in your own healing.

Through my exploration into healing my own trauma and working with grief I have found eight key elements that are vital in helping to move forward and embrace the joy of living. It can be a tough process but I have learned one simple fact: there is nothing wrong with admitting I am a work in progress and I am not perfect. *You* are a work in progress and *you* are not perfect, and that is completely fine. Acceptance of who you have become and who you are at the present moment will bring you inner peace. I hope you will find the eight key elements useful on your healing journey.

1. Make your intention to heal clear to the universe and, more importantly, to yourself. Use the following affirmation: 'I am ready to heal.'

2. Focus your attention: do not allow distractions or self-destructive talk. Take a few cleansing breaths to focus your mind and direct your attention on what you need to address in order to ease the healing process.

3. Keep an open heart: always keep your heart open to welcoming love and joy no matter how hard it is.

4. Release everything that does not serve you in your quest for healing. Use the following affirmation: 'I release any negative energy that is obstructing my healing process. I invite only positive energy to bless my healing process.'

5. Commit to undertaking the healing work every day. Use the following affirmation: 'I commit to always do what it takes to heal every single day.'

6. Have hope: inculcate a desire for change, as it will keep the flame of trust burning.

7. Love: love is our blueprint for life. Always go back to love.

8. Have faith: faith is knowing deep inside you will be all right. You may never be complete, but you will still be doing just fine.

Every one of us is a work in progress. Always be gentle to yourself and to others.

What is slow grieving and why is it important?

Grief will always be a part of your life. It often comes uninvited and can take you by surprise with a shockingly fierce grip at the most unexpected moment: in the middle of the supermarket, on a commute to work or as you sit down for a meal. You desperately try to fight back the tears and you take a deep breath and put on a brave face. 'Not now,' you whisper to grief and you keep repeating this scenario over and over again, hiding your grief and pushing it away every single time because you need to be brave, but grief needs time and space. In order to heal you need to grieve and mourn. There is no way around it; you have to go through it and take the storm full on. It is scary and unimaginable, but you need to follow this process.

I promise that over time grief will become less overwhelming. Slowing down to grieve means you give it all the time it requires from you with self-love and compassion. You will listen carefully with your heart and with every breath until every facet is familiar and every dark aspect is exposed to the light. Gradually, grief will become an old friend who visits you occasionally, staying for an hour or two or a whole day but when it eventually leaves there will be no devastation or deep, fresh wounds. Instead, there will be a glimpse of renewed faith and hope and even a sense of lightness as you move with steady steps along your healing journey.

I invite you to slow down and take a deep breath to separate yourself from the chaos and demands of daily life. Imagine a vast garden that needs painstaking effort and a large amount of determination for it to flourish and reveal its hidden beauty, then imagine you are this vast garden. This is what you will be creating when you slow down, take a deep cleansing breath and grieve. You are attending with tender loving care, patience and self-compassion to every corner of your emotions. Nothing will be left untouched or uncared for. While taking care of your emotions you are also paying attention to your physical and spiritual needs.

The heartache, deep sorrow and despair that have become part of your life will gradually make way for transformation. As you slow down to grieve fully and mourn your loss you unveil within the depth of your soul a new meaning of life. Grief has many layers, but as you remove layer after layer you will finally discover a new revelation that otherwise would have remained unseen. Whatever the revelation is, embrace it and work with it rather than against it.

I invite you to explore the art of slow grieving through the self-care practices in this book. Each practice has been carefully chosen to address topics that may arise during the grieving and healing process.

THE ART OF GRIEVING

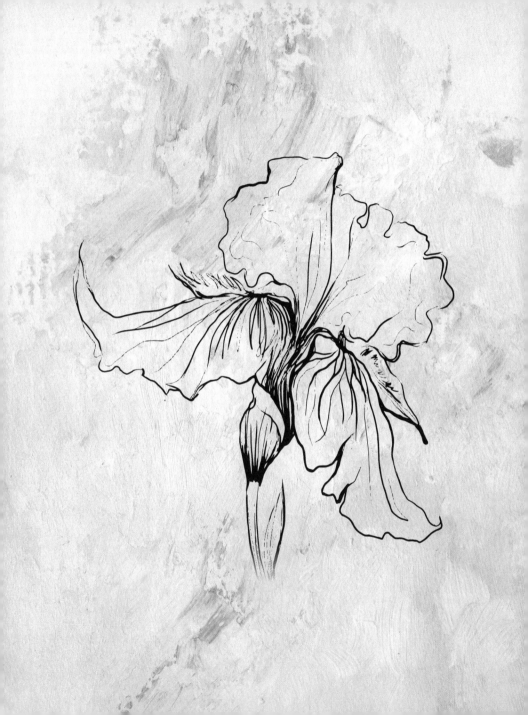

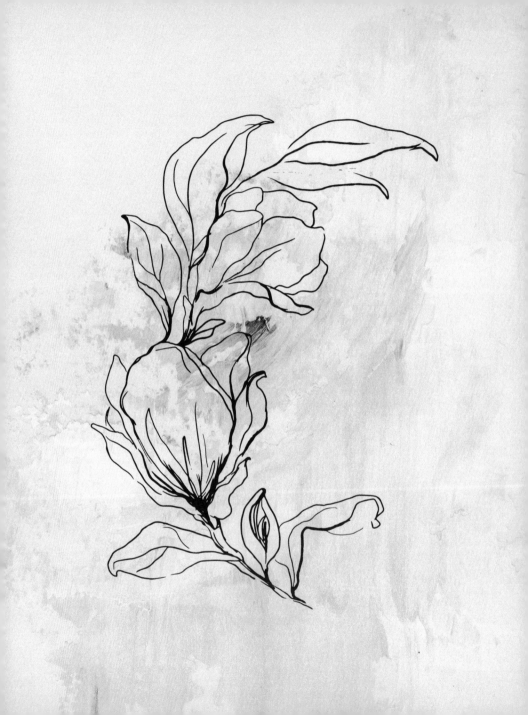

2

Using rituals for self-care practices

supercharge your healing process

Undertaking rituals is a beautiful way to embrace your grief. When you see the word 'rituals' it may invoke images of religious rituals in an exotic foreign land or even rituals associated with cults. Perhaps you think rituals can only be performed by spiritual leaders. However, these days the word is used in a much broader sense and commonly to describe a practice that is done on a regular basis. 'Beauty rituals' and 'self-care rituals' are some of the terms that have emerged in modern culture.

Your body and mind often disconnect following the emotional trauma of loss as your mind is busy trying to make sense of the recent event while your physical and emotional bodies are actively dealing with the loss, the trauma of which creates changes you didn't expect or were prepared for. The feeling of disconnection or being out of sync can last for months or even years. Any activity or practice done with intention on a regular basis – a ritual, in other words – has the remarkable potential to reconnect body and mind.

The sadness you feel is crushing and the impact it has on your health and well-being can be challenging. Left untouched, the emotional and physical toll will eventually become apparent: it will seep into your day-to-day life, affecting your home environment, social and work life and your relationships. The emotions associated with grief are not bad emotions; they are necessary emotions that need to be expressed and channelled into a less destructive force. When emotions are acknowledged and tended to with all the love and compassion you can gather it can bring new insights into your own strength, your ability, your potential and even, dare I say, a future you did not know was possible before. Rituals provide a safe haven along with a well-defined platform to honour grief and to mourn your loss with reverence, empathy, compassion and love.

As you actively take part in a ritual you are engaging with your grief within the safety and carefully woven structure it provides. The reality and pain of your loss, no matter how difficult it is, become less daunting. You have a platform upon which you can safely explore the changed person you have become, find new meaning in life and recognise the people around you who are supporting you during your time of need and pouring love into those relationships.

The ritual way: from brokenness to wholeness

The ritual way is a path I encourage you to explore because it gives grief the time and space it requires from you without taking what little energy you have left. Through rituals you can delicately weave emotional trauma, mourning, sorrow and healing into the rich canvas of daily life. Rituals bring you back to wholeness as they contain all the powerful ingredients for transformation, so utilising them is an effective means of unlocking your very own healing potential.

We all possess healing abilities and a ritual is the perfect ally. In our fast-paced lives, which require us to move at an equally fast speed and very often at the detriment of our healing and well-being, the ritual way can provide an oasis of calm in which we can process a loss and fully attend to our emotions.

The beauty of rituals is simply the invitation of positive energy regardless of religious beliefs. Rituals are part of everyday life: they can be the little things you do on a daily basis or elaborate ceremonies. Getting up every Sunday morning and pouring yourself a delicious cup of coffee to enjoy in peace while still wearing your pyjamas is a ritual. The modest cup of coffee with its inviting fragrance becomes a vessel of pure positive energy, a sparkle of joy and a feeling of warmth on what could otherwise be just another day.

Rituals are essential for the healing process as they embody all the principles of healing: keeping an open heart, making your intention clear and focusing attention along with release, hope, love and faith and, last but not least, a commitment to do the healing work. When you engage in a ritual it needs to be meaningful to you so you can harvest its true potential. A ritual is an eloquent expression of deep intentions that in turn engage your mind in a powerful yet delicate manner. The humble act of engaging in a ritual can help shake off any negative thoughts in your unconscious mind and help uplift your mood and lighten your heart. It helps you hold on to hope, love and faith when you feel lost in the chaos of grief.

When the pain of grief is too overwhelming we often build a dense wall around us, toughening our hearts and letting no one inside. We use all kinds of diversion techniques in order to disengage from the pain or push it far away.

The key to healing from deep sorrow is to move with the pain and never against it. Imagine a small vessel in the vast ocean moving with the ups and downs of each wave, big and small, as it keeps moving steadily towards the harbour. This vessel is you, taking each big or small wave of grief in your stride as you slowly but surely move forward. You must listen to the pain of sorrow and find what it is trying to tell you so you can transform the pain into something positive and less destructive. In order to transform the pain of loss you need to be creative with it, as the pain that comes with deep sorrow needs movement. There is no better way to help pain move with and through your body and soul than through a ritual.

Key element of rituals

Below are listed the key elements to a ritual. Bringing together these simple steps when you are performing a ritual will help you immensely on your grieving journey and may bring a gentle boost to your healing process.

- **Gift of presence:** make a conscious effort to be entirely present during the ritual, not only physically but emotionally and spiritually as well. Set aside a time and place to carry out the ritual, choosing a time of the day when you will have no distractions and not feel rushed.

- **Symbolism:** symbols play a big part in bringing meaning to a ritual. They can be important objects in your unique story of life, love and loss such as flowers, candles, photographs, pieces of jewellery, crystals or even aromatic scents such as a burning incense.

- **Intention:** I cannot stress enough that the key piece to any ritual is intention, which is what gives the practice its distinct healing spark and meaning. Before you perform any ritual, ask yourself these simple questions: what is it you want to happen, and what do you need right in this moment? Perhaps you want to feel calmer or you simply want to move forward on your healing journey. Whatever the intention is, be clear in your mind. Take a few cleansing breaths and hold the intention in your mind before you move on to actually performing the ritual. Once you have set your intention the ritual will feel more authentic.

- **Order:** any ritual needs to have a beginning, middle and end. The beginning should be gentle, then the ritual will pick up pace before a slow closing component.

- **Open heart:** a ritual is merely going through the motions if you do not bring with you an open heart. Be open to any emotion and thoughts that may arise during the ritual; accept what is without judgement, love and compassion and with an open heart. Do not be afraid to pour your heart and soul into your ritual.

- **Spirit:** in ancient Chinese script the heart is described as the place where spirit dwells. If you are performing a ritual with your heart you will inevitably bring a spiritual element to the ritual. Each individual will have a different idea of what 'spirituality' means, so just go with what resonates the most with you. It can be acknowledging there is a divine presence bigger than us or a pure light or a god. The spiritual element to the ritual will over time bring the spark that may have been missing within you, the spark that brings joy and meaning to life.

The steps for performing a ritual

The first step in performing a ritual is *choosing the right space*: your sacred space, a dedicated space for the sole purpose of doing your rituals. Space is everything when it comes to performing a ritual. It needs to be a place where you feel at ease and safe and removed from chaos and possible distractions or interruptions. It needs to be a place where you can turn inwards and invoke your higher self as well as uncovering your inner wisdom and inner strength. A dedicated space for your rituals will focus your mind and, over the course of time, gather energy and sacred vibrations, all the positive energy you can instantly feel as soon as you enter the space. In times of great stress, sadness, loneliness and agitation your sacred space will provide solace and will be somewhere you can find refuge, take a deep breath and ground yourself.

Choose a private space that can easily be transformed into an oasis of calm. It can be indoors, or if you are lucky enough to live in a warm climate an outdoor space would also be perfect. If you live in a small apartment, a corner of a room is more than adequate. Allow yourself to be creative with the space you have available. Most of all, the space you choose should be visually inviting: a colourful cushion, a soft delicate blanket or throw, a bright rug and fresh flowers will immediately engage your mind and invite you to indulge a few minutes of your time in a self-care ritual.

Once you have chosen your space the next step is to *create your peaceful haven*. Allow yourself to be in the flow of pure creativity and not feel restricted in your choices. If you are on a tight budget and cannot afford to buy special items, one easy solution is to gather things you already have around your home and create your unique sacred space. With something simple as the right colour palette you can create a space that is appealing to your senses and spiritual needs.

Colours have different religious and cultural meanings. Some believe it is not necessarily the colours themselves that have special meaning but rather that we have given special meaning to them. Other people believe colours have potent energy and as such emit vibrations that can be harvested for specific purposes. Regardless, we can safely say colours can influence our moods: some colours make us happy while others make us feel sad and withdrawn.

Colour therapy is a fascinating subject when it comes to healing, so here is a brief overview of some colours and their meaning for you to explore:

- **red** represents vitality, passion, enthusiasm and love
- **yellow** represents wisdom and may reduce mental confusion
- **orange** is often associated with creative energy and joy
- **green** represents nature, life and balance
- **blue** may be used to represent spirituality and peace
- **purple** represents sorrow, peace, spirituality and creativity
- **white** represents innocence, light, purity and mourning
- **black** represents strength, death, power and mourning
- **gold** is often associated with strength
- **silver** represents peace
- **pink** is often associated with love and happiness.

You may have your own interpretation of colours and some colours may hold special meaning for you. Take a moment to explore these and which colour palette or colour combination best suit your needs, your sacred space and your intention.

The next crucial phase of your ritual is *bringing healing vibrations to your space* with a unique piece straight from the heart. I love using art as a form of expression, and creating intuitive pieces with watercolours or pastels can be a healing practice. There is nothing more calming and soothing to the soul than tapping into your intuition and allowing your piece of art to gently take shape and reveal itself. You do not need to be an artist to create an intuitive piece; it requires only your intuition mixed with your creative flow and, above all, complete detachment from the final result. When it comes to grieving and healing you are a blank canvas, and just like an intuitive piece you should not be attached to the outcome. You are perfect just as you are.

Supplies to consider gathering for your intuitive piece could include a piece of cardboard or paper thick enough to handle watercolour; a watercolour palette; paint brushes; a jar of water to clean your brushes and mix your paint; and a tray to mix the paint with water.

This simple activity is about letting go of fear, judgement and attachment to the end result. It is about allowing yourself to be in the moment, in complete flow, and allowing the piece to reveal itself. There are no mistakes here; rather, each colour forms a welcome base for the next layer of colour. Just as the healing process has many layers, so too does the painting process: each step you take on your healing journey forms the base for the next step. The painting process also serves as a gentle reminder that healing is messy and, just like the piece of art you are creating, your grief and healing are unique to you.

When your intuitive piece is ready, hang it proudly in your sacred space. It will be your reminder of the steps you are taking each day towards your healing, a reminder that messiness and imperfection are part of the grieving and healing process.

The next phase of your ritual is *creating your altar*. Every sacred space needs an altar or centrepiece, as it is the heart and soul of the space. When you come to your sacred space to sit in silence or pray you will direct this at your altar. An altar can have many items, each of which will depend on your spiritual and religious beliefs. I love creating an altar with crystals, shells and flowers, as these items remind me to always see the beauty of the world.

You can choose items that hold special meaning for you in your time of grief. If no special items come to mind straight away, that is perfectly fine. As you start gathering and choosing items for your altar you will intuitively be drawn to certain items. If you would like to keep your altar minimalistic, this is also perfectly fine: it is your space and should feel right for you.

Your sacred space should hold positive and inviting energy, so the final critical phase of undertaking a ritual is *cleansing your sacred space*. Clean your space on a regular basis with locally sourced cleansing products if you can. Clear the space regularly of all negative energy using sage, palo santo or incense. Open the windows and curtains to allow the fresh energy of sunlight or moonlight to flow in. If you have an outdoor space, sweep the area regularly and keep it free from weeds, dead leaves, twigs and dirt.

If you love essential oils you can use them to invite fresh, vibrant energy to a recently cleansed space. Add 10 drops of your favourite essential oil or oils to a diffuser. Start with five drops and then increase the quantity if you need to. My favourite essential oils to use are jasmine, rose, lemon, orange, ylang ylang and may chang.

Finding your flow: self-care menus

You may find it easier to have a plan in place to help you get into the habit of performing rituals if you are new to them. Creating a self-care menu is a stress-free way of finding your flow and embracing the grace of rituals. Even if you are experienced at undertaking rituals, you may still find it helpful to have a menu. Life can be chaotic, and it is easy to neglect your practice in difficult times.

Below are several examples of self-care menus. Plan your menu in advance for the week or month ahead depending on your needs.

Monthly self-care menu

Ritual for mind and soul:	Ritual for emotional health:
Ritual for physical health:	Ritual for spiritual health:

Daily self-care menu

Day of the week	Ritual to be performed
Monday	
Tuesday	
Wednesday	
Thursday	
Friday	
Saturday	
Sunday	

The key to healing
from deep sorrow is
to move with the pain
and never against it.

3

Mind and soul rituals

slowing the pace

Sometimes we can be so busy trying to keep our heads above water we forget to stop and listen to what we really need. Emotions guide behaviour, and sometimes we need to create the space in our busy minds to listen deeply so we can adjust our behaviour and respond to situations with compassion and love.

● *Inner compass ritual*

For the inner compass ritual, sit comfortably in a quiet spot where you will be undisturbed.

Place both of your hands on your heart space and gently close your eyes or lower your gaze. Take a few deep breaths and ask yourself: which emotion is calling your attention today? Listen deeply to the messages of your inner knowing. Take your time; feel and listen.

When an emotion comes to the surface attend to it with love and kindness. What can you do now to help ease this emotion?

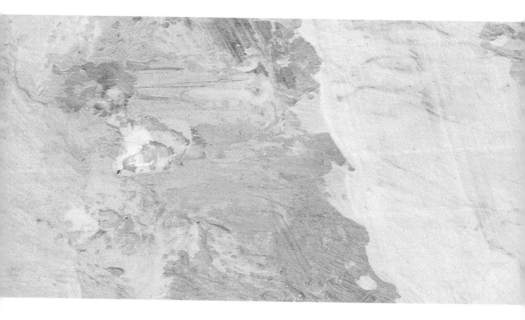

THE ART OF GRIEVING

❚❚ *Ocean ritual*

I was born on a tropical island and the ocean fascinated me from a young age. I have always felt its powerful energy: the sea, the beach and the salty breeze have cleansing effects on the mind and soul and the ability to dissolve heavy emotions and bring peace to your heart and spirit.

If you are fortunate to live by the ocean, go for a walk along the beach. Choose a quiet spot, and inhale the salty air. Allow the energy of the ocean to wash away your sorrow.

If you live far away from the ocean (and even if you live close by), listen to recorded wave sounds while you meditate or just before you go to sleep at night. This can be very soothing, especially if you are facing challenging times.

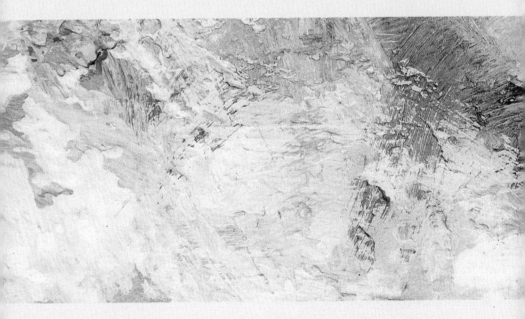

● *Prayer ritual*

Prayer is a powerful healing ally that restores hope as well as faith. When the world around you seems to collapse, a prayer will help to ground you, offer a moment of solace and shift your mindset.

Your sacred space is the ideal spot for a prayer ritual. Light a candle on your altar and, if you like, add some incense. Take a moment to ground yourself and set your intention, then close your eyes and say a little prayer straight from the heart. Complete this ritual with a grateful heart.

You might like to try this cleansing prayer:

> *May I be cleansed of all negative emotions and energy. May my healing path be blessed with strength, courage, trust and love. May love flow through me, healing my body, mind and soul. May I always feel the warmth of love as I allow the gentle flow of life to pull me in.*

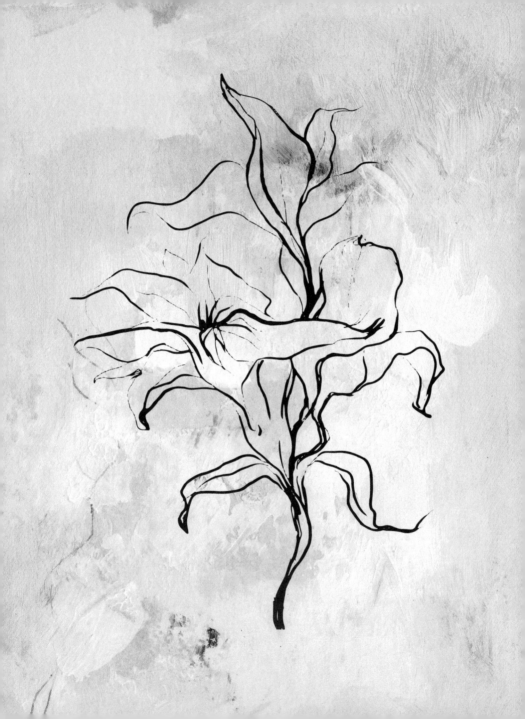

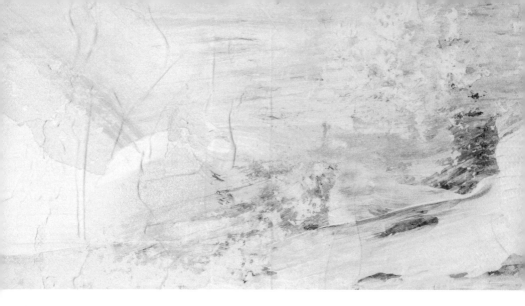

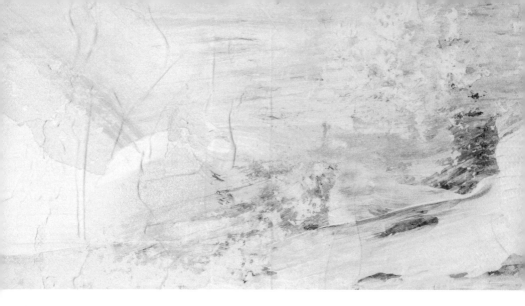 Ⓥ *Meditation ritual*

A powerful method for healing your mind, body and spirit, meditation restores your body's energy as well as helping you to feel more grounded. The mind craves stability in times of great sorrow and uncertainties and, as a way of coping, fills the silence and the void with chatter and chaotic thoughts. The mind can do one of two things: try hard to make sense of the chaos and the loss or try to numb the emotions. As you continue on your grieving journey, meditation can provide solace in the midst of chaos.

Meditation will provide your mind with enough time and space to allow you to feel without being pulled into the chaos of your emotions. It can provide the shelter your soul is longing for. Slowly, as you build your practice and meditation ritual, thoughts will become clearer. You can even feel the stress caused by heavy emotions becoming less severe.

Facing grief requires courage, faith and endurance, and meditation offers a wonderful tool that can work very well alongside other healing methods and therapies. The key to meditation is to go into it with a sense of curiosity rather than expectation and allow it to unfold. It requires discipline and a willingness to practise it regularly, so instead of approaching it as yet another exercise on your busy schedule or another task on your endless to-do list, make a commitment to explore meditation with a sprinkle of inquisitiveness and an open heart. Look upon meditation as a gift you deserve: you are worthy of inner peace.

If you are new to meditation, start with the following simple meditation ritual.

Choose a meditation space – your sacred space is ideal – and a time of the day that works best for you. Early morning is generally perfect, but explore your options to find which time of the day or night suits you the most and fits in with your schedule.

Sit with your spine straight and your chest open, using a meditation cushion for comfort. Allow your whole body, including your muscles and bones, to be free from tension. Allow your shoulders to sink towards the floor and soften your facial muscles. Rest your hands on your lap with your palms facing upwards.

Soften your gaze or close your eyes, and take a few cleansing breaths to clear your mind. You may wish to use the rhythm of your breath, a sound or even a sensation in your body to anchor yourself in the here and now and accept, feel and experience each moment.

You may find that internal chatter occurs and thoughts come cascading in; this is completely normal. When you notice you have been lost in chatter or thoughts, simply acknowledge it without judgement and allow the thought or distraction to flow away from you as you exhale. Anchor yourself again in the present, in the here and now.

Practise the meditation for around 10 to 15 minutes to begin with. As you become more familiar to meditation you can gradually increase your practice to 30 minutes.

(v) *Earth energy meditation script*

You may wish to add this short meditation that will connect you with the nurturing and healing energy of the earth to your ritual. Your sacred space or outdoors in nature in a private, quiet spot would work very well.

Sit restfully on the ground, using a cushion and blanket for extra comfort. Make sure your spine is straight, your chest is open and your hands are resting on your lap with the palms facing upwards.

Gently close your eyes or lower your gaze and slowly bring your attention to your breath, feeling its rhythm and your chest rising and falling with each breath. As you breathe out, release any tension in your body. Release and relax more with each breath; as your body relaxes so does your mind. All distractions and thoughts slowly fade into the distance and you feel calmer and at peace.

As you relax more it feels as though the base of your spine is sinking deeper into the ground. You feel connected to the earth's energy. As you exhale, allow all negative energy and all negative emotions you may be holding inside your body and mind to move freely along your spine towards the base of your spine and finally travelling into the earth, where they will be absorbed and dissolved.

Take a few minutes to visualise the emotions and thoughts moving through your spine and into the earth each time you exhale. When you are ready to move on, visualise your body being free of all negative energy.

You are now ready to receive the healing and nurturing energy of the earth. Imagine or sense this energy beneath you. Continue to sense this beautiful healing energy moving upwards towards your spine and rising all along it, expanding and wrapping you in a soft blanket of support and love. You feel at peace and spiritually grounded.

When you are ready to close this ritual, gently bring your attention back to your surroundings. Move your toes and fingers, and when you are ready slowly open your eyes.

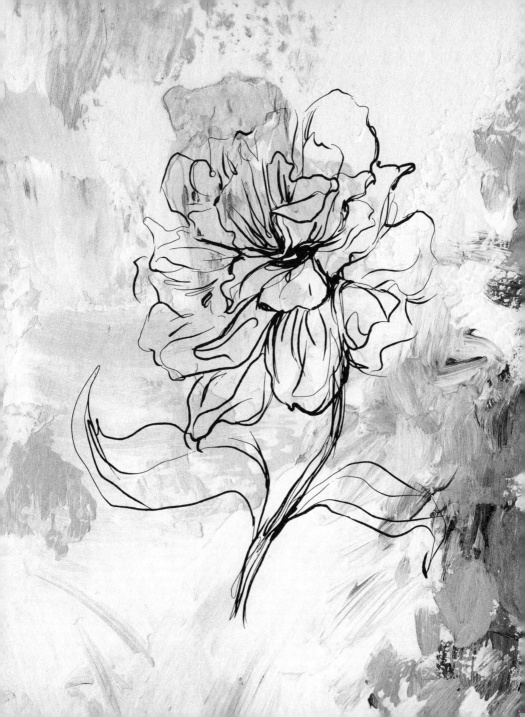

Ⓥ *Healing heart meditation*

This short meditation will connect you with the universal love that surrounds you. All you need to do is be aware of it so you can access its essence.

Sit restfully on the ground or on a chair, using a cushion and blanket for extra comfort.

Gently close your eyes and slowly bring your attention to your breath, feeling its rhythm as the air enters and leaves your lungs and your chest rises and falls with each breath. As your body relaxes your mind follows and starts to relax. All thoughts and distractions fade into the distance.

Imagine or sense a soft pink cloud surrounding you and gently enveloping your entire body with its gentle mist. It feels reassuring, peaceful and relaxing to be surrounded by this soft pink cloud. Feel its pure loving energy: it is compassion in its purest form, it is empathy in its purest form and it is love in its purest form. You feel in harmony with everything within you, and you feel in harmony with everything outside of you.

As you continue to follow the rhythm of your breath you become aware of every single organ and every single cell in your body pulsating in harmony with the loving energy surrounding you. You feel deep peace. Place your hand on your heart space and breathe nine times into it. Bring your hand back to your lap, and breathe in and breathe out.

When you are ready, gently bring your awareness back to the room. Move your toes and fingers and slowly open your eyes.

All is well. This loving energy is always present whenever you need it.

VII. *Diamond mudra ritual*

The diamond mudra, also known as *vajrapradama mudra* meaning 'unshakeable trust', is perfect for when you feel overwhelmed by difficult emotions and other challenges. The mudra awakens the heart energy and, by doing so, enhances trust and self-confidence and erases self-doubt and hopelessness.

To perform the vajrapradama mudra your body must be relaxed. You can sit comfortably in the lotus pose or, if you prefer, in a prone position or stand.

Take a few deep breaths to help you relax before you begin, then interlace your fingers with your thumbs facing upwards towards your collarbones. Bring your hands over your heart space and rest them on your chest, positioning your elbows wide. Your fingers and hands should be soft. Close your eyes and breathe, and connect with your heart energy. Stay there for as long as you want.

The vajrapradama mudra is an affirmation practice. Over time, you will start to notice and feel its benefits and the changes within you.

Ⅷ *Dream ritual*

Dreams can sometimes be a reflection of your inner anxieties and fears and at other times a mirror of your hopes. Following a loss, you may experience vivid dreams that leave you feeling shaken and recurring dreams are also common.

Recording your dreams in a dream journal may help you reflect and make sense of your dreams, which are very personal and have their own meaning and significance. Keep your dream journal and a pen by your bedside, then as soon as you wake and before you step out of bed quickly jot down your dream to capture its essence.

Make some time to revisit your dream journal. Sit comfortably in your sacred space and read what you have written down. Pause and reflect. You may not see any significance or deep meaning straight away, but your subconscious works quickly. Over time, you may see the true meanings behind your dreams.

THE ART OF GRIEVING

Ⅸ *Soul dance ritual*

Grief can sometimes feel as though it is stuck deep inside your body and nothing you do helps to lift your mood. Movement can shift your mood and uplift your spirit, and even bring a spark of joy into your heart and soul.

Put your favourite music on and start moving with the rhythm of the beat. Move your body slowly to start with and then allow yourself to be free. Dance around the room until you feel uplifted and your mood has improved.

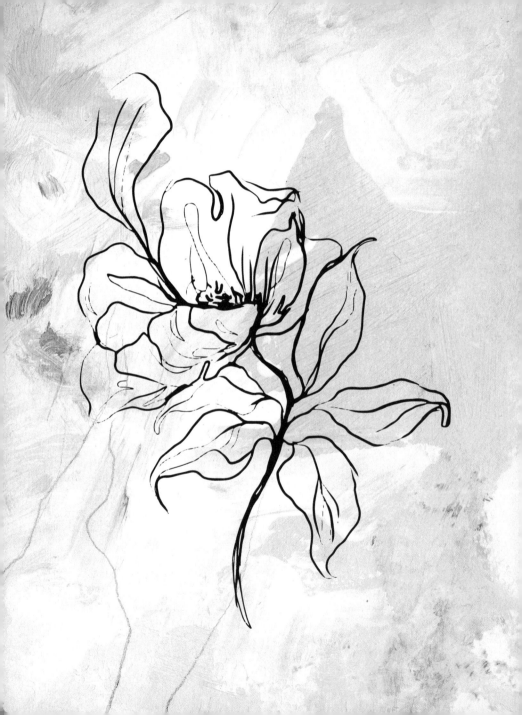

4

Release rituals

set yourself free

Letting go of negative energy and emotions, the past, toxic relationships and anything that no longer serves you is a powerful step on your healing journey. Release rituals offer you the space to find strength as you embrace the painful pieces of your story and let go of the pain. By clearing the emotional clutter you actively create space for inner peace and joy.

① *Release negative energy ritual*

Following a loss you may feel negative energy from your distant past starting to creep up, perhaps from relationships that ended badly or even from past losses. All of this unresolved energy may become compacted into one overwhelming wave of negativity. This ritual is an invitation to release all the negative energy that is not contributing to your well-being.

Add some fresh flowers to a vase and light a candle in your sacred space to create an area of beauty and serenity, which will help you to feel more at peace. Make yourself comfortable and place your hands on your lap. Take a few cleansing breaths to release any tension in your body.

When you are ready to begin, close your eyes and say the following in your mind:

> *Today I make the choice to release all negative energy and past hurts and disappointment. I am ready to embrace joy and happiness. I am strong; I am loved.*

Repeat this as often as you like.

When you are ready to complete the ritual, slowly open your eyes and snuff out the candle or, if it is safe to do so, let it burn completely.

⑪ *Forgiveness ritual*

Forgiveness of self and others is a powerful habit that will restore peace in your heart and mend broken relationships, both of which are essential for your healing journey.

Light a candle: white for purity or pink for love. Take a few cleansing breaths and release any tension in your body.

Close your eyes slowly and bring your attention to your breath, allowing your heart space to open with each breath. Feel, sense or visualise a beautiful light in your heart. You are at peace.

Bring each person who needs your forgiveness to your mind, and for each one silently repeat:

I forgive you. I release you, and as I release you we are energetically freed from each other. I wish you well. I forgive you.

To conclude this ritual, make sure you also forgive yourself. Silently repeat:

I forgive myself: the things I have done, unkind words I have spoken, the resentment I have felt. I release. I let go. I forgive. May I find peace.

Snuff out the candle or, if it is safe to do so, allow it to burn out.

⦿ *Releasing anger ritual*

A loss of any type can leave you feeling angry, which is a normal emotional response after a loss. However, if the anger is not dealt with it can cause health-related problems both short term and long term. If you're feeling overwhelmed by anger, practise this ritual at least once a week.

Create a relaxing atmosphere with a few drops of sandalwood, pine or lavender essential oil in an aromatherapy diffuser. Make yourself comfortable in your sacred space.

Take a few deep breaths to release any tension in your body and bring yourself to the here and now. Place your left hand on your heart space and slowly close your eyes.

Ask for the gentle guidance of love and compassion to help you through this difficult time. What does your anger feel like: is it a tightness in your throat, or is it a heavy sensation in your chest? Wherever the sensation is, observe it from afar. Don't engage with or question the sensation; just take note of the physical manifestation of the anger.

As you breathe, imagine sending love and compassion to this sensation. With each breath, continue to visualise sending loving kindness until the sensation starts to fade or feel lighter.

When you are ready to complete this ritual take a few deep breaths, and as you exhale visualise the last remaining sensation floating away from you. Slowly open your eyes.

Make a gentle mister to ease anger by adding 10 drops of lavender, which brings comfort and emotional balance, to 100 ml of distilled water in a spray bottle. Don't shake to mix. Instead, place the lid on the bottle securely and swirl the bottle gently first clockwise then anticlockwise. Give the bottle a little swirl before each use. Spray the mist in front of you and walk through.

Ⅳ *Releasing anxiety ritual*

Anxiety is a natural response to grief. You may feel fearful about the future or apprehensive about the next step you should take.

When you feel anxious and pulled into a spiral of fear, take a moment to ground yourself. Add 10 drops of essential oils to a diffuser; equal parts of angelica root (for grounding) and orange (for joy and self-confidence) work well together. It is best to avoid using angelica root if you are pregnant. When working with essential oils it is good practice to start with less and increase the amount if needed. Kick off your shoes, spread your toes and feel the ground underneath you. Take a few deep cleansing breaths and soften your tensed muscles.

Use the following affirmation or create one that resonates with you:

> *I am resourceful. I am capable of turning things around. I am in complete control of my mind and my life. I am fearless.*

Tip 1: you may want to carry a talisman in your pocket or purse to give you extra support or wear a pendant that holds special spiritual meaning for you. Wearing a crystal such as amethyst or clear quartz will help you to stay calm and grounded.

Tip 2: add movement to release anxiety. Qigong is perfect for relieving anxiety. You can create your very own ritual by incorporating qigong to the early morning, which is described in Chapter 8.

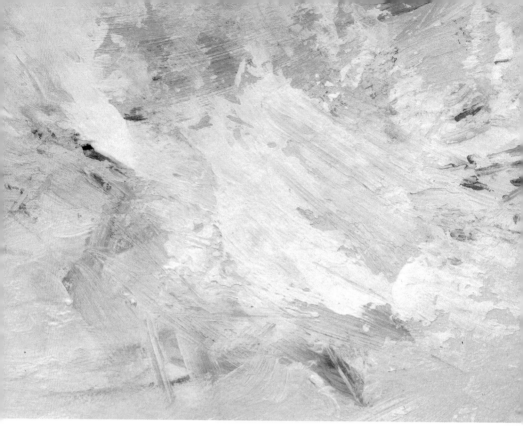

Ⅴ *Reclaim your power ritual*

You may feel powerless or helpless after a loss and during the grieving period that follows, and these feelings can linger for weeks, months and even years. You may find it difficult to make decisions or follow through with your plans and dreams because deep inside you have lost the self-confidence you once had.

Reclaiming the kind of power that enables your spiritual growth and helps you live your life to its full potential will supercharge your healing. When you reclaim your power you cut all the strings that tie you to the feeling of hopelessness. As you let go of the disabling belief that you are powerless you can finally release all the other negative destructive beliefs that may have crept into your subconscious. As you reclaim your power you reclaim your right to stand in your truth, recognising what is important to you and trusting your ability to make the right decisions.

The power that connects you to feeling whole again is within you.

Practise this ritual outdoors if you can for the best result, although your sacred space would be a good substitute.

Stand with your bare feet hip width apart, spreading your toes and allowing your feet to be in full contact with the ground. Move gently from side to side and back and forth until you feel comfortable. Loosen your hips and knees. Close your eyes and take a few deep breaths.

Bring your attention to your feet and feel the places where they are touching the ground. With each breath, allow your feet to sink deeper into the ground. Visualise, feel and sense this connection with the earth. Like a tree standing tall and strong, so are you. Despite the storm here you are. You are as strong as ever; you are powerful and have never lost your power.

Repeat silently and as many times as you desire:

> *Today I reclaim my power. I am a powerful being. I am whole again. I am complete.*

When you are ready to close this ritual take a deep breath as you bring your arms above your head. As you exhale bring the palms of your hands together and lower your arms towards your chest, your hands in a prayer pose. Place your hands over your heart space and slowly open your eyes.

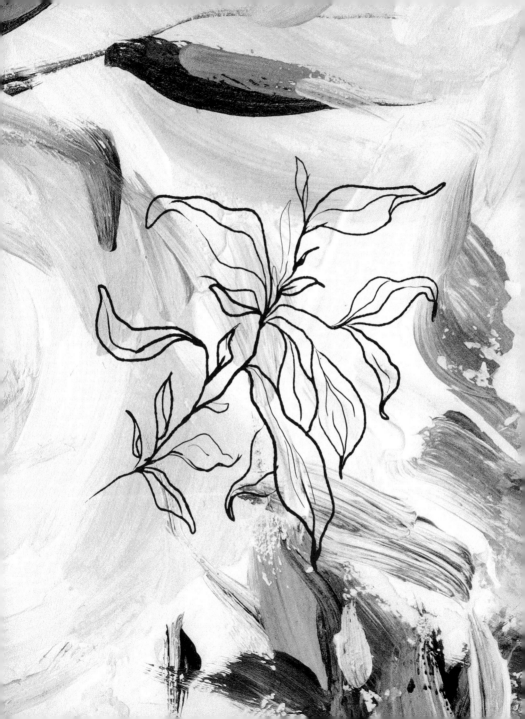

5

Gratitude rituals

building resilience

Gratitude is absolutely not being grateful for the loss or pain you are going through, nor is it saying good things happened because of this. Rather, it is recognising wonderful things happened despite the loss. It is about getting the mind to see through the pain, and it is about giving yourself the space to see and be grateful for some if not all of the positive things that surround you despite your terrible, heartbreaking loss. It is about creating a shift in your mind that is almost like moving through clouds.

Once your mind slowly makes the shift you will gradually become aware of the new perspective you may have of life, the new relationships you may have forged since the loss and the love of your family and closest friends. Beyond the pain and sorrow there are blessings always happening within and around you. Once you make the space to actually see them in your mind and sense them in your body you will start to feel lighter as the heavy dark clouds of deep sorrow gently lift.

This is healing. When we acknowledge our blessings we create a vast positive shift in our energy and vibration. This positive vibrant energy in turn makes us more receptive to the positive energy around us.

To see the blessings of what loss and grief have brought to your doorstep you must first wear grief. By this I mean you must acknowledge the presence of grief in all its ugliness – not because you are a brave being but because there is no other choice. Facing the storm head on is the one and only way to get to the other side of grief and to the subsequent healing beyond.

Gratitude keeps your heart open. You can use 6 to 10 drops of essential oils in a diffuser as an extra boost to balance and open your heart chakra; choose one or make a blend from the following essential oils:

- *rose*: invites in love and compassion
- *bergamot*: opens your heart
- *neroli*: invites in love
- *lemon*: invites in love
- *Roman chamomile*: promotes peace, love and compassion.

Enjoy the fragrance as it fills your home and at the same time balances your heart chakra.

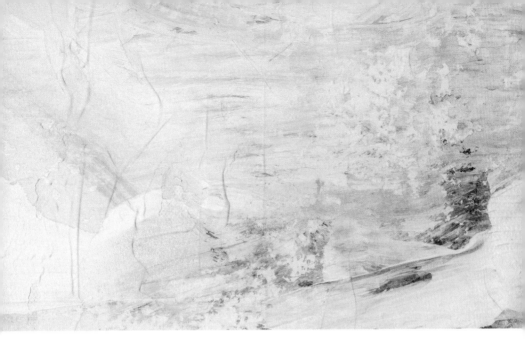

⬤ *Small blessings ritual*

This ritual, which will allow you to embrace your blessings in whichever form they choose to manifest themselves, can be performed towards the end of the day.

You will need a medium-sized tray, a white (for purity) or pink (for love) candle and some crystals. Choose a crystal you feel most drawn to from the following: rose quartz (for love), malachite (for calm and emotional balance), amethyst (for grief, calming the mind and enhancing your aura) or moonstone (for compassion or to remove energy blocks).

You can add some personal items such as a piece of jewellery, a figurine or a pebble or shell you have gathered from a beach walk. The item you choose needs to have a special meaning to you.

Place the candle in the middle of the tray and arrange the crystals you have chosen and your personal items around it to form a circle, which is a representation of the love energy that is always present and never ending. It also represents the circle of life, a constantly moving circle.

Before you light the candle, take a few cleansing breaths. Clear your mind of all the troubles of the day and set your intentions. Take a moment to contemplate the flame and watch it dance in front of you; feel its warmth permeate your heart.

Bring your attention to the here and now. Release all tension in your body and take a deep breath as you feel your body sinking into relaxation. Feel the softness of your body connecting with the inner stillness of your mind.

Bring forth in your mind a blessing and, when you can see it clearly, sense it in your heart. As you begin to feel it in your heart place your left hand on your heart space. Give thanks with love.

If you cannot think of any blessing you can silently say the following words:

I give thanks today for each and every blessing that surrounds me even though in this space and time I am unable to see or feel them in my heart. I know the blessings are here and I am grateful.

Continue for each and every blessing and for as long as you wish.

When you are ready to end your ritual you can either allow the candle to burn out if it is safe to do so or snuff the flame. Make this ritual part of your daily or weekly routine.

⑪ *Cultivating a grateful heart ritual*

It can be so hard to keep your heart soft and be grateful because you may feel there is nothing to be grateful for: you have lost so much and it hurts. However, keeping a grateful heart helps to change your mindset and your whole vibe from negative to positive. You attract the energy you put out there. Turning things around is the hardest thing you will have to do, but you can start slowly.

Take a few minutes away from the chaos of life and sit quietly in your sacred space. Light a candle if you wish. Take a few deep cleansing breaths and bring your attention to your heart space. This ritual requires you to listen with the heart.

Name one thing you are grateful for today. Perhaps someone you love dearly is still here with you and you get to spend another day with this person. Perhaps you are grateful you are in good health. Keep searching, and once you have found it give thanks:

I am grateful for . . .
I am thankful for . . .

As you practise this ritual over time you may want to include more than one thing you are grateful for. You can include as many as like.

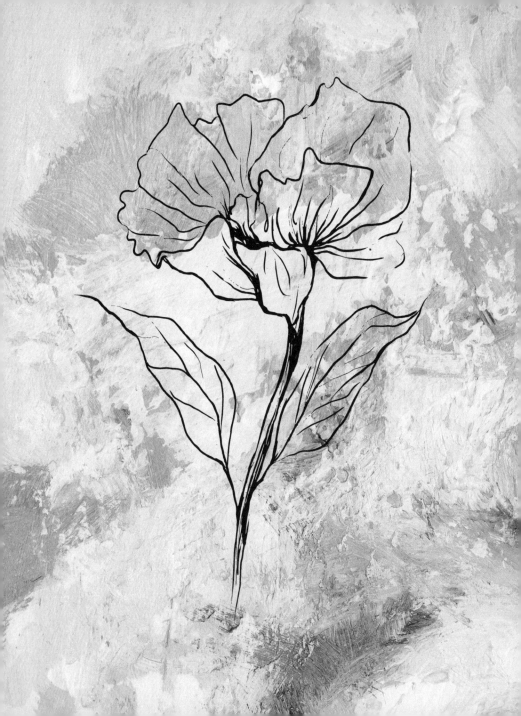

6

Water rituals

soul cleansing

The ritual of bathing goes back thousands of years and has its roots in many cultures, religions and traditions around the world. The act of pouring water over the body is believed to have purifying and spiritual meaning. Water has the ability to induce relaxation, with its properties having a deep effect on the physical as well as the spiritual body.

In India, for example, worshippers gather on the banks of the Ganga River to perform rituals. Also known as Ganga Ma (Mother Ganga), it is believed the waters of the river can purify as well as protect worshippers from danger and evil. In Bali, in the sacred water of Tirta Empul (the holy water spring), worshippers engage in bathing rituals. In Mauritius, the Grand Bassin or Ganga Talao is a sacred lake for worshippers of the Hindu faith. In almost every region of the world there is a water spot known for its healing properties, such as the hot springs in Iceland and Hungary.

The healing and soothing properties of water can be utilised in your own home.

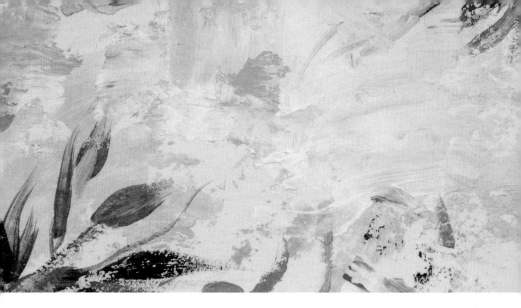

⬤ *Salt bath ritual*

Salt is well known for its cleansing properties and has been used and is still being used across the world in many civilisations and cultures. It can cleanse auras and absorb negative energy from your energy field as well as promote relaxation by releasing muscle tension.

When you feel weighed down by negativity or your energy feels a bit off you can add a handful of salt to your bath water. Clean and cleanse your bathroom and open the window and door to allow fresh air to come in.

Set your intention as you fill the bathtub with hot water. Light a couple of soya candles and place them around the bath. You can add crystals to bring the grounding energy of the earth. Add a handful of salt to the bathwater. I prefer using rock salt as it does not contain any toxins or pollutants. Allow the salt and water to work their magic and visualise being cleansed of all negative energy as it is neutralised by the salt.

Close this ritual with a grateful heart, giving thanks to the elements you have used during it: air, fire, water and earth.

⬤ *Essential oils salt bath ritual*

You can also make a healing salt bath by infusing the salt with healing prayers and essential oils.

Cleanse your space before you begin making the salt. You can reserve items only for the purpose of making special blends for your rituals, treating everything you use with love and care. Each item should be treasured and pleasing to the eye, as these items will bring beauty to your healing work. I love using delicate china, antique pharmacy bottles and colourful ceramics to make and store my salt blends. I also like to give thanks to the plants I use in my blend as it helps me to stay connected to the wonders of the world and all the beautiful gifts it has to offer.

Use any of the following essential oils:

- **Geranium** carries the vibration of Mother Earth, embodying feminine energy. It offers comfort while healing from the pain of loss and can bring tranquillity and balance.

- **Lavender** offers the subtle protective love of Mother Earth. When deep sorrow weighs heavy on your heart and bears your spirit down, lavender will gently lift your spirit. It provides comfort, calmness and acceptance.

- **Marjoram** offers shelter from the chaotic world and calms the senses. It brings peace, balance and perseverance on your healing journey.

- **Melissa** brings understanding and compassion when words cannot express what is being felt by your heart, mind and body. It offers spiritual guidance as well as bringing renewed energy, strength, acceptance and joy.

- **Neroli**, with its calming and relaxing scent, can reduce stress, depression and anxiety and relieve insomnia.

- **Rose** is a reminder of unconditional love and the gift of giving this love freely, including to yourself. It awakens your heart chakra and eases grief, and brings love, acceptance, harmony and purity.

- **Ylang ylang** offers protection, warmth and heavenly awareness. It brings emotional support to your heart and mind on your healing journey.

Important note: *if you have sensitive skin, omit melissa and ylang ylang. If you suffer from low blood pressure omit ylang ylang.*

Before you prepare your blend set your intention firmly.

Use a small amount of base oil such as almond oil to mix the essential oils before adding them to the salt. In a glass bowl, combine 2 tablespoons of salt with 12 drops in total of any of the essential oils above. Allow the mixture to infuse for 24 hours and store in an airtight glass jar.

Add a healing prayer to your blend. You can write the prayer on a piece of paper and place the jar on top of it or you can recite the prayer while making the blend:

> *May I be held in love and compassion.*
> *May the light shine upon me as I wander*
> *through the shadows of deep sorrow. May*
> *I show loving kindness towards myself.*

May I find the courage and strength to persevere. May my heart awaken again to the joy of life. May I find peace in my heart and acceptance on my healing journey.

Toss around 1 tablespoon of the infused salt into warm bath water and allow the special blend and the soothing effect of the water to provide you with comfort and healing.

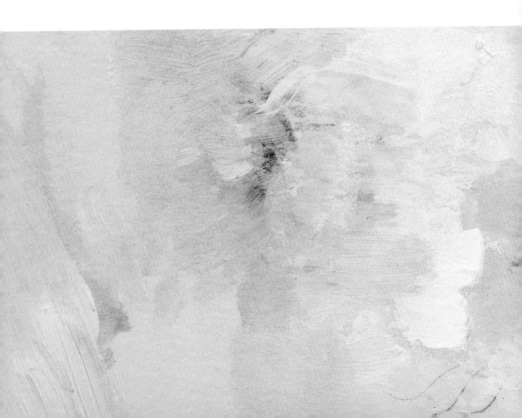

◉ *Rock salt foot soak ritual*

After a hard day you may feel overwhelmed by an array of emotions and that you are not doing enough to heal your sorrow or you are not enough. The world seems just too much, almost to the point of being unbearable. You may feel disconnected within, your mind and body moving at difference paces, as well as feeling disengaged with the outside world.

If you experience any of these feelings, this rooted in spirit foot soak is an essential self-care ritual. A quick and easy way to relax and ground yourself firmly in the here and now is to fill a foot basin with warm water, add a generous amount of rock salt and soak your feet, then take deep breaths to relax and feel grounded.

If you would like to add some extra healing power to your foot soak, try this foot soak recipe. You will need a small jar with a lid, 2 tablespoons of rock salt and four drops of angelica, clary sage or white spruce essential oil. Add a crystal to supercharge your foot soak if desired; rose quartz, amethyst, lapis lazuli, citrine and mookaite are all good choices.

Note: avoid these essential oils if you are pregnant or suffer from epilepsy.

Before adding the essential oil to the sea salt in a glass bowl, mix it first with a little almond oil. Fill the jar with the mixture, add the crystal and seal the jar. Allow it to infuse for 24 hours before using it in your foot soak.

⒧ *Mystic mugwort tea bath ritual*

Mugwort (*Artemisia vulgaris*) is a lunar herb that is commonly used for women's health discomforts as well as digestive problems. On an energetic level, mugwort opens the energy channels in your body, removes blockages and encourages flow.

Mugwort is a nervine (nerve tonic) and therefore has an effect on the nervous system. It can induce deep relaxation and remove stress from your body and protect your heart energy and liver energy, making it a perfect herb when going through a significant transition in life. As a messenger plant it helps you to connect with nature as well as promote lucid dreaming.

Seventeenth-century herbalist Nicholas Culpeper said mugwort had the ability to dissolve sorrow from the heart. He also referred to mugwort as being connected to Venus and Leo, with Venus symbolising love and Leo symbolising strength and courage when facing sorrow. Sometimes, love, strength and courage are needed to help you to move forward.

If you are using fresh mugwort fully fill a 1 litre Mason jar, and if you are using dried mugwort fill the jar halfway. Pour hot water into the jar, cover it and let the mixture steep for four hours.

Run a warm bath. Beautify the bathtub by placing crystals of your choice and candles around it. Create a welcoming space of pure calm that is inviting to the senses.

When your bath is ready, strain the mugwort before adding the tea to the bath. As you do this, thank the medicinal plant for its wisdom and healing properties. Relax in your bath and enjoy the benefits of this beautiful healing herb. When you are ready to get out of the bath, visualise leaving all that no longer serves you behind in the water. As you remove the bath plug and watch the water drain away, visualise everything you are wanting to let go of being neutralised by the loving energy of the earth.

Important note: *do not use mugwort if you are trying to conceive or are pregnant.*

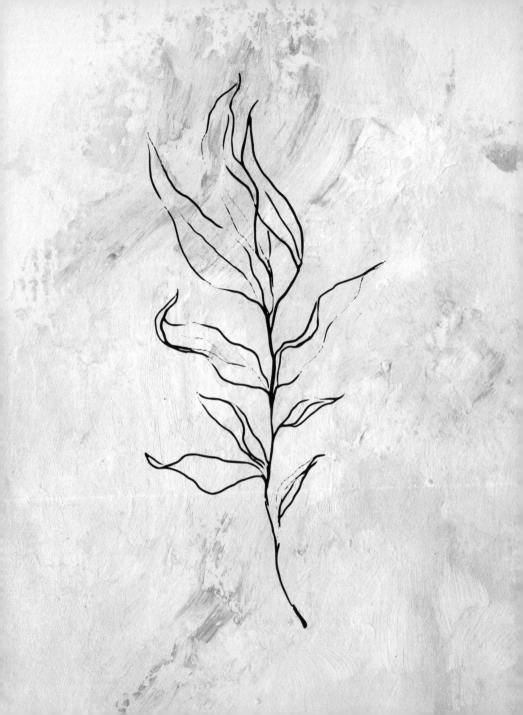

7

Stillness rituals

finding solace

One of the greatest gifts of all is the ability to receive ourselves with love and compassion and in the complete absence of judgement, self-blame and guilt. We are often our own worst critic, and when we let ego take control our focus is shifted to the outcome, which clouds our vision from turning inwards and recognising our potential and ultimately moving forward on our healing journey.

Take a long moment to truly be there for yourself without judgement. Offer yourself the space for reflection and eventually self-healing will emerge. When you create internal space it paves the way for transformation. You have within you the gift to turn things around even if this task looks impossible right now. Spending some time alone allows you to tune in to and listen to your needs. Grieving is chaotic and messy. Those around you, although well-intentioned and supportive, may unknowingly hinder your grieving process. It is a good practice to carve out some time to listen to your own needs, to recharge your spirit, to reflect and to heal.

❶ *Solace ritual*

Set aside at least 20 to 30 minutes for this ritual and find a comfortable space away from potential distractions, because what surrounds you externally can affect you internally. Your sacred space at home could be the ideal spot. Choose flowers, soothing music, a clean, clutter-free room and anything else that awakens a sense of calm, which will help you to feel more grounded.

Before you begin, clearly set your intentions. You are here to create space within and you can only do this if you are prepared to receive yourself with love and compassion and without judgement, self-blame and guilt.

When you are ready, take a few cleansing breaths and clear your mind of any distracting thoughts that may interfere with your ritual. Now is a good time to let go of any lingering negative thoughts that may have haunted you in recent times. Let go of expectations and take a moment to refocus on your intention. In this space there is room only for love and compassion, to see yourself exactly where you are without judgement and to listen to and hear yourself with a charitable heart.

Ask yourself what needs your tender loving care today and what emotion, particular challenge or worry needs your love and compassion right now. Listen deeply and breathe. Be gentle with yourself; you are a wise being and know how to proceed. Remind yourself of this: you too deserve the love and compassion you give to others.

Silently state the following affirmation:

I am worthy of love and compassion. I am healing beautifully each and every day.

🄚 *Unwrapping the new you ritual*

Grief changes you. You are a different person to the person you were before the loss. There is this part of you which is missing. Holidays and birthdays will never be the same again. Discovering your new identity and who you are now after the loss is challenging. However, if you keep yourself wrapped up in the busy-ness of life, you will struggle to get to know the new you.

I recommend doing this ritual at least once a month. You can start with one hour and slowly build up to a whole day. This ritual is particularly helpful after a divorce or break-up.

Choose a favourite spot. This may at the beginning be your sacred space and later as you practise this ritual more, you may want to venture away from home and find a place where you will feel comfortable to spend a few hours. As you spend time by yourself, you will gain new insights of who you are and thoughts will become clearer.

Take notes to capture your thoughts. Before going on your retreat have a clear intention. You may want to add a specific goal for your healing as well.

Always start this ritual with a short breathing exercise combined with a short meditation. You may wish to light a candle. The colour of the candle can bring focus to your intention. For example; a white candle is for purity; a pink candle is for love including self-love, a red candle is for passion in a relationship, a purple candle is for wisdom and a silver candle is for feminine energy.

Complete this ritual with a grateful heart. Give thanks for the insights and thoughts which have emerged during your time in stillness.

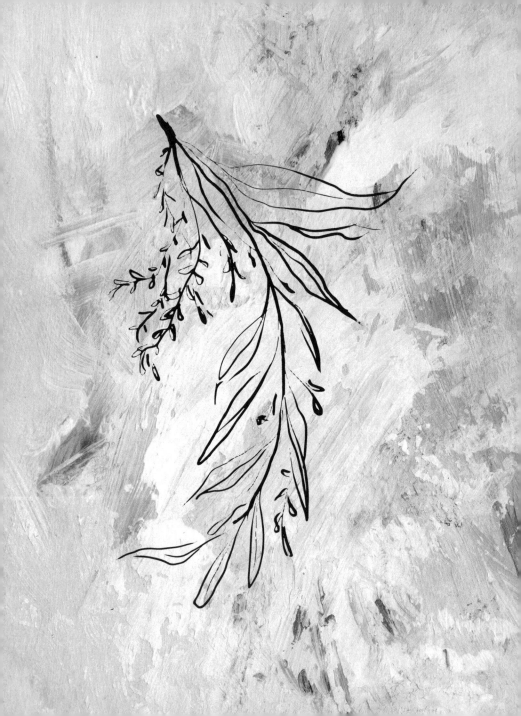

8

Nature rituals

restorative gifts of Mother Nature

Nature is a great healer and a sacred gift you can access whenever you feel overwhelmed and stressed. Spending any amount of time in nature can bring inner peace and allow you to appreciate the mystery of life. As the time of the day changes or a new season makes an entrance so does the landscape; it is a gentle reminder that nothing is permanent and everything changes, and that despite this everything is in perfect balance. When you are out in nature and notice the colours, sounds and fragrances surrounding you it immediately engages your mind and provides a peaceful haven where you can rest your broken heart.

1 *Early morning ritual*

At daybreak when darkness is gradually being replaced by light it symbolises transformation and new beginnings. This is a very personal and sacred time.

For this ritual you need to get up just before sunrise when everything is still dark and silent outside. Sit comfortably facing east. You may close your eyes for a moment and take a few deep breaths to centre yourself. When you are ready, slowly open your eyes and look at the horizon. As the first light breaks observe the change in colour and listen to the sounds around you as the world wakes up to this new day. Be very aware of the sensations you are experiencing.

You can add an affirmation, blessings or a poem of your choosing to welcome the magic a new day brings. When you feel you are ready to end the ritual, give thanks to this day with a grateful heart.

THE ART OF GRIEVING

▌ *Sunset ritual*

The sunset ritual is an invitation to slow down. As the sun disappears over the horizon it is a reminder to let go of everything that could not be resolved today and to give gratitude for everything that was accomplished. Shake your hands, arms, legs and hips, letting it all go. Visualise, sense and feel all the worries and frustration of the day falling from your body. Shake it all off.

You can do this ritual just before going into the shower and allow the water to do the last final cleanse. Take a moment to complete the day with a grateful heart.

⦿ *Silent walk ritual*

The spirit of beauty has been discussed for centuries by shamans and philosophers. We and all flora and fauna are living reflections of the beauty of the universe. When you wake up to the beauty and sacredness of every plant and living creature and the sun and the moon, negative energy and emotions cannot stay for long. They start to melt away.

This ritual invites you to respond to the world around you with love. When you allow the beauty of the world to enter your inner space and allow every cell in your body to mirror this beauty, all negativity that may have been affecting you will slowly melt away.

Turn off your phone to minimise distraction and take a silent walk in nature. See, sense and feel the world around you with your heart and from a place of love and intense curiosity. Take a moment to stop and observe everything around you, from the trees, the birds, the insects and the flowers to the sky and the clouds above you. Practise seeing with your eyes and feeling and sensing with your heart.

Take a deep breath and invite the beauty around you to go within.

ⅳ *Remembrance garden ritual*

Creating a remembrance garden at home can bring you closer to the one you lost. It is a beautiful way to honour your grief and fills any void you may be experiencing. Working with the soil and planting seeds can be a deeply soothing experience to the soul. If you do not have an outdoor space, a corner of a balcony with plants in pots or inside your home can work just as well. You will need some seeds to plant and gardening tools.

As you get ready to create your remembrance garden, take a few deep breaths and set your intention. It can be that you are dedicating this plant corner in memory of a loved one or you are dedicating this space in nature as a quiet space to honour your grief. As you begin to work the soil and plant the seeds, say a little prayer or a poem. Take the time to acknowledge your sorrow and give it the space it needs in this moment.

You may wish to silently repeat the following affirmation:

> *As I take care of the plants I give the same attention to my grief. As I take care of this garden I give the same love and kindness to my broken heart. As I take care of this garden and plants I remember and honour you.*

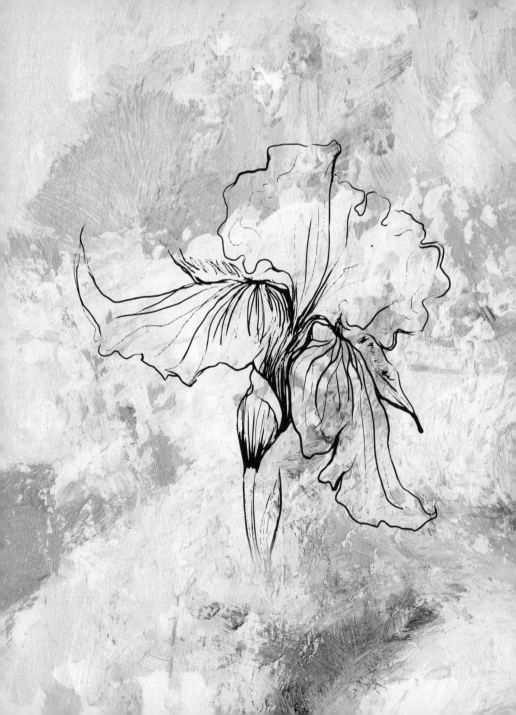

9

Love rituals

love is everything

Love is both the source and the remedy to our sorrow. The seed of grief is love and the seed of healing is love. Without love there is no grief, and without love there is no healing.

Love + loss = grief
Grief + love = healing

Sorrow and love have their roots in the heart space. Sorrow is constricting, whereas love is expanding. This duality dwells in the same space and a large portion of healing is learning to live with the duality. Feeling the constriction of sorrow and at the same time allowing love to flow freely and expand through your entire body then pouring it out into the world takes both time and dedication.

When you are grieving you may unconsciously close your heart to love, as it is a normal reaction to protect yourself from further emotional harm. Your instinct is to shut down and safeguard your fragile heart.

In the face of extraordinary challenges love is often the only answer; it is a potent remedy. When you strip away your insecurities, self-doubt, beliefs, career, assets and body, what is left? When you take a deep look within and beyond the layers, beyond the superficial aspects of what define you as a human being, you will see love; it is your blueprint. Love is the beginning; love is the end; love is all the in-between spaces. Love is everything. Love connects you to your soul and to every other living creature on the earth.

When you speak from a place of love and act from a place of love you connect with the divine, with god and with spirit. When you connect to this pure energy called love you allow your deep knowing and wisdom to guide your every step.

Give love. Receive love. Be love. If love has been lacking in your life lately, reclaim it now. You are worthy of love and your life purpose is to share it with those around you.

One of the very first steps towards love is to invite it into your home, which is your sanctuary and a reflection of your inner space. Decluttering your home can be a symbolic act of decluttering your inner space. As you get rid of unused or broken items around your home you create a positive, fresh and renewed flow of energy and a space of calm, a true sanctuary where you can unwind.

Bring nature inside your home with plants and fresh flowers. As you take care of the plants you reconnect with your nurturing instinct and eventually love will start to flow again in your heart. If you love crystals, place a rose quartz in a room where you tend to spend most of your day such as your living room or home office. Hang a picture portraying a loving, peaceful scene.

Colour matters in a home. Add a sprinkle of red to bring passion back into your life. A red vase or a red decorative object will bring love and ecstasy into your space.

Practise the art of giving: donate items you no longer use to charity or volunteer for a charitable organisation to bring a feeling of abundance.

Practise the art of receiving: be open to receiving love in any form, whether it is a compliment or a gift, to make love grow stronger. Love is like a magnet: love attracts love.

❶ *Self-love ritual*

This ritual is an invitation to open your heart again to love. Self-love is not about being self-centred, nor does it feed the ego; it is pure love that nurtures the soul.

Learning to be tender and kind to yourself is a key element in the healing process. Loving yourself again after a loss of any kind can be difficult, as the burden of guilt and self-blame may weigh heavily on your soul and you may feel that you do not deserve to be loved. Self-love opens the door to self-acceptance. When you practise self-love you begin to accept where you are and the reality of the loss and your new identity.

THE ART OF GRIEVING

Self-love brings a welcome sense of peace to your body and soul. As you practise the self-love ritual your heart will begin to soften. Your inner knowing will start to gently steer you towards the path of love over and over again. Loving yourself fiercely is the best remedy for a broken heart. It compels you to say a big 'yes' to life and to new beginnings.

Sit comfortably in your sacred space or outside in nature, somewhere peaceful where you will be undisturbed and can take all the time you need. Take a few deep breaths and relax and allow yourself to sink comfortably in your seat. Silently repeat the following prayer:

May I accept and love myself. May I cultivate a forgiving and loving heart. May my heart only know love. May I be free of all things that do not serve me in my healing journey. May I find inner peace and happiness. May I choose love. In difficult times, may I always find my way back to love.

Repeat the prayer as many times as you desire.

Tip: rose quartz is the love crystal, so carry one in your pocket or purse or wear a rose quartz pendant close to your heart.

⓫ *Fall in love with yourself ritual*

There are five simple steps to the fall in love with yourself ritual:

1. Write down 10 things you love about yourself.

2. Treat yourself: go out for a meal in your favourite restaurant, soak in a bubble bath, visit a local place you have always wanted to visit, take up a hobby you've always wanted to do but have always found an excuse not to start or take an afternoon off and indulge in a new novel or movie. The list is endless!

3. Turn your phone off and go for a long walk in nature, which has a healing effect on the soul and helps you to reconnect with yourself.

4. Every morning, look at your reflection in the mirror and silently repeat to yourself:

> *'I love myself and I am worthy of love, joy and happiness.'*

Smile, because you are beautiful!

5. Practise meeting yourself exactly where you are without judgement.

⦿ *Love pick-me-up spritzer*

For this simple spritzer, which I found in one of Valerie Ann Worwood's aromatherapy books, you will need an essential oil such as lavender, neroli or rose otto or any other oil that is associated with love, a stainless steel pot with a lid and a 150 ml spray bottle.

Pour 150 ml of water into the pot and add a few drops of essential oil. It is better to start with less and experiment with the quantity that feels good for you; you may also want a more subtle fragrance. Start with one essential oil then later you can mix several essential oils together and make your own blend. As a reference you can start with 18 to 20 drops of essential oils in total. It is always a good idea to keep a notebook of your recipes for future reference.

Tightly cover the pot and bring the water and oil to a boil. Remove from the heat and allow the mixture to cool, then place it in the refrigerator for 24 hours with the lid still on. After 24 hours, scoop out whatever drops of oil you can see floating on the surface; you can use these in a diffuser to avoid wastage. Pour the remaining water in a spray bottle, label and use around the room whenever you need a little more love in your day.

ⅳ *Love ritual*

Record what you hope to gain from this ritual in your journal, including your hopes and wishes. Perhaps you would like to be more open to love or would like to invite more love into your heart, especially if you have been having difficulty connecting with your loved ones or you would simply like to feel and sense the sweet fragrance of love in your life again.

For this ritual you will need to prepare the herbal incense, which can be found in Chapter 11. If you do not have the time to make the incense you can use rose incense instead and skip the candle part.

Take a few cleansing breaths and light a pink or soya candle. Sprinkle some of the incense on the candle, and as the incense burns breathe in the aroma. Pay attention to how you feel and release all the tension in your body as you breathe out. Take a moment to focus your mind as you continue to breathe in the aroma. Visualise the smoke sending loving energy to your entire body. Open your heart with each breath and allow the aroma to wrap you with love.

Silently repeat the following affirmation as many times as you feel you need to:

> *I am loved. I am love. I receive love. I give love. Love is my path. Love heals my sorrow. I am open to love. I remain open to love.*

After the ritual, take a moment to reflect and capture your thoughts in your journal. What did you feel or sense during the ritual? How did you feel before and after it? When you look at your wishes and hopes from performing this ritual, did you come close to achieving them? Are they within your grasp?

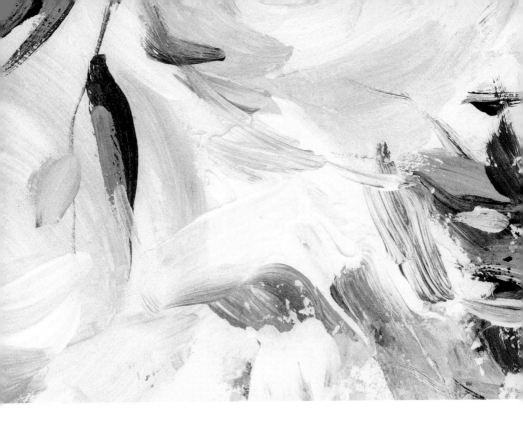

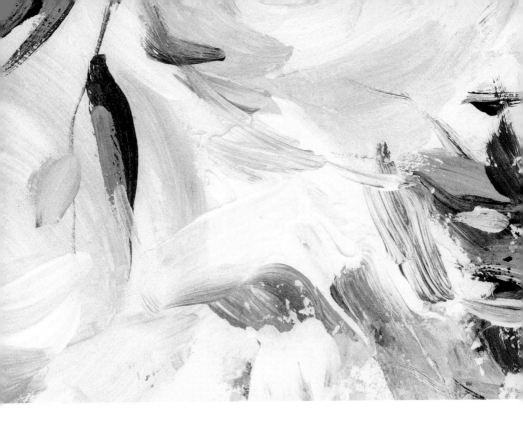 Self-compassion ritual

This ritual helps to cultivate self-compassion, an essential part of your healing journey. If you have been particularly hard on yourself this ritual will soften your heart and allow you to let go of self-blame and judgement. As you perform this ritual, over time you will feel more grounded.

Take a moment to bring a recent event that requires self-compassion to your mind. Do not allow yourself to be pulled into the details or the emotions associated with the event; simply bring it to your conscious mind. You may be hurt, disappointed or ashamed or feel betrayed. Acknowledge your emotions without judgement.

Take a few cleansing breaths to release any tension in your body, allowing it to flow away as you exhale. When you are ready, bring your hands into a prayer pose.

Silently repeat the following prayer as many times as you feel you need:

May my heart be filled with loving kindness. May I always find strength to forgive myself. May I accept myself exactly as I am and where I am. May I always return to love.

When you are ready, place first your left hand then your right hand on your heart space. Take a few slow, deep breaths and allow every cell in your body to flow with the renewed positive energy you have just created.

Perform this ritual whenever you feel you need some loving kindness. You can close your day with this ritual for a peaceful night's sleep after a particularly overwhelming day.

Tip: create a compassion altar in your home as a daily reminder to be kind to yourself and to always treat yourself with loving kindness. Choose a space where you can set up a small altar, adding candles, incense sticks, crystals and flowers. You can add a deity of your choosing. If you love working with crystals, rose quartz, peridot, amethyst and malachite are good choices to invoke compassion. Once your altar is set up in your chosen space you can say a little prayer to invite in only the purest and highest energy.

Ⓥ *Loved one ritual*

As you navigate your way through the journey of grief you may unintentionally have built thick walls around you to protect your grieving heart. As you slowly emerge from the fog and numbness you may feel a sense of guilt for having neglected the ones you love and cherish. It is never too late to rebuild relationships and reconnect with family members and close friends. Nurturing healthy relationships is a self-care practice and is part of your healing journey.

You will need pieces of coloured paper cut into heart shapes, a pen, a memo board and pins. On each piece of paper, write the name of a loved one. Secure the hearts on the memo board with pins and place the board somewhere readily visible as a reminder to nurture the relationship you have with each person on it. Every morning as you drink your cup of tea or coffee, pick a name from the board. Give them a thought, a thank you for being in your life or for something generous and kind they did for you. Send this person a message or, if you like the old-fashioned way, send a letter, card or small gift via the post.

Complete this ritual with a grateful heart.

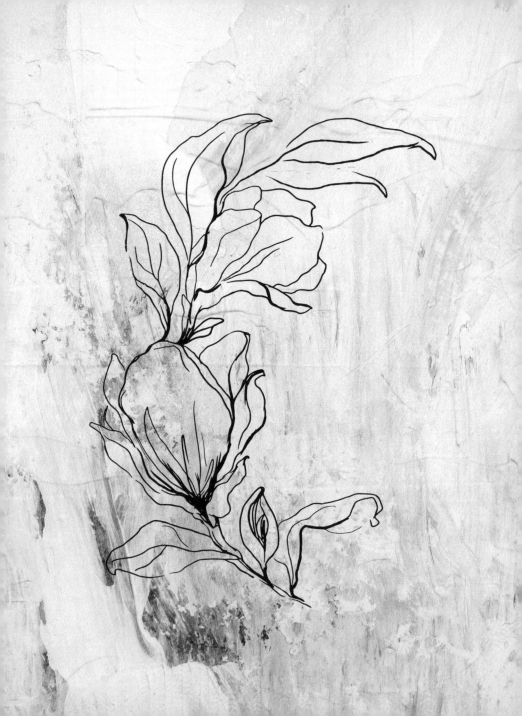

10

Peace rituals
cultivating calmness despite the chaos

In spite of all the pain and the obstacles you have experienced or may still be experiencing you deserve to feel whole again. Sometimes in order to gain peace you have to let go of the things you cannot change and take a different path or find a solution to a problem. Cultivating peace requires courage and daily input so you can work towards achieving it. You are more likely to feel peace when you are engaging in activities that bring you joy or are living a life that aligns with your core values. However, life circumstances and negative emotions can creep in and disturb your inner peace, so when this happens it is good to remind yourself that it is only temporary and that you are in control of your inner peace at all times.

● *Peaceful heart ritual*

According to Chinese medicine, the heart is the emperor of all organs and is the seat of the mind. It is the king of joy and rules with wisdom, compassion, love and peace. Regarded as being a fire element, the heart gives life and movement, is the organ associated with awareness, feelings and thoughts and connects you with nature and unconditional love. A peaceful heart allows you to go with the flow and not be burdened by fear and instability.

For the peaceful heart ritual your sacred space will be the perfect spot. You may choose another spot where you will be undisturbed and can take all the time you need to perform the ritual.

Light a white candle for purity or a pink candle for love. A tea light can work just as well; the choice is entirely yours. You may wish to add incense to this ritual; rose for love or jasmine for purity are both good choices.

Begin by setting your intention for a peaceful heart and the ability to welcome more joy into your life. When you are ready, make sure you are sitting comfortably and have a blanket or shawl over your shoulders to keep yourself warm.

Place your hands on your lap with the palms facing up. Take a few cleansing breaths to release any tension in your body and let go of mind chatter. Allow the thoughts to flow away from you and into the distance, then return your attention to your breath.

Notice the rise and fall of your chest with each breath. Imagine, feel or sense your breath flowing in and out of your heart space. Sense how your heart space feels without judgement. Continue to imagine or sense your breath flowing in and out of your heart space.

As you continue to breathe in and out of your heart space, imagine it getting lighter and expanding with each breath. Visualise a door at the centre of your heart space, and as you continue to breathe imagine the door gently opening with each breath. Continue until the door is completely open.

As you continue to breathe, imagine a ray of light entering your heart space through the open door. Feel abundant love, compassion and peace pouring in with the light ray and fill your heart with this beautiful energy.

When you are ready, place first your left hand on your heart space and then your right hand. Welcome love, compassion and peace into your heart and allow this renewed energy to flow throughout your body with each breath. Take your time; there is no rush.

When you are ready, slowly return your awareness to your surroundings. Move your toes and fingers and open your eyes. You may wish to remain for a little while longer in complete silence. Pour yourself a warm cup of tea and enjoy a moment of peace.

❚❚ *Peaceful sleep ritual*

Emotional trauma and grief can adversely affect the rhythm and quality of your sleep. You may suffer from insomnia, or have difficulty falling asleep or wake up in the early hours of the morning and be unable to get back to sleep. Sleep is the body's natural mechanism to rejuvenate cells, and the quality of sleep is just as important as its length. Poor sleep can affect your concentration and have adverse effects on your daily routine. A lack of sleep can make you irritable, frustrated and exhausted. You may become more prone to bouts of anger, and depression may set in. Your body particularly needs adequate rest during the grieving and healing process.

The peaceful sleep ritual is best done in your own bed made up with fresh sheets. Fluff your pillows, give your bed cover a good shake and add an extra blanket if it is needed.

Make yourself comfortable in the prone position with your head and neck well supported by pillows. Place your arms alongside your body with the palms facing up. Take a few cleansing breaths and adjust yourself until you are perfectly comfortable.

Slowly close your eyes. Scan your body and release any tension, starting from the tips of your toes and gradually working your way up until you reach the crown of your head. Each time you feel or sense tension breathe into it, and as you breathe out release and relax a little more.

Bring your attention back to your breath. Feel the air on the tip of your nose as you breathe in and out, and stay with this sensation for a while. Feel the air entering your nostrils and filling your lungs with air. Feel your chest rise and fall with each breath. Allow all worry or negative emotion to flow away from your body as you exhale. See them fading away and disappearing into the distance: beyond the walls of your bedroom, your house and past your neighbours' houses until they completely disappear.

Follow the rhythm of your breath and allow yourself to melt into deep relaxation. Everything you need physically, emotionally and spiritually is being taken care of. You can completely let go and embrace the gift of a deep, peaceful sleep.

◉ *Head massage ritual*

Grief can leave you feeling exhausted, but despite being overly tired you may find you are unable to relax and drift off to sleep. Your mind seems to be in overdrive. If you are experiencing difficulty falling asleep or having vivid dreams, the head massage ritual is a perfect bedtime ally.

Touch is a wonderful and powerful healing art. Have you ever had a massage that was so relaxing you felt every muscle tension had magically melted away and you left the massage table floating on a stress-free cloud? This is the magic of healing touch. If you are unable to book yourself a relaxing massage, outlined below is a self-massage ritual to help you find the deep relaxation your body is craving for.

Self-massage is a divine habit to cultivate: your own hands can bring comfort and alleviate certain ailments you may be experiencing. This ritual is a perfect addition to the peaceful sleep ritual above that uses various acupressure points on the head to calm the mind and reduce stress as well as easing insomnia.

Find a quiet spot where you can be undisturbed for at least 30 minutes such as your meditation space or bedroom. You may want to sit on a yoga mat supported by cushions or at the edge of your bed; the key is to be completely at ease.

Yin tang or 'hall of impression' is an important point in qi gong, 'impression' in this sense meaning 'inner visions'. The yin tang acupoint is located midway between the medial ends of the two eyebrows, similar to the third eye chakra. Yin tang helps with headaches, calms the mind and relieves anxiety, mental restlessness and insomnia.

Place your index and middle finger on yin tang. Massage in a circular motion either clockwise or anticlockwise, whatever direction feels best for you. You may want to close your eyes or lower your gaze. Continue to massage for about five minutes and keep breathing nice and slowly, following the rhythm of your breath.

Tai yang or 'great sun' must be treated with the utmost respect as it is a sensitive point and only a very light touch is required; just enough pressure to move the skin is usually enough. Just as with yin tang, tai yang also calms the mind and relieves headaches. It is located at the tender depression of the temples.

Use the soft padding of your index and middle fingers. Use your right hand for the right temple and left hand for your left temple. Gently move your skin upwards then, following a clockwise motion, downwards and back up again in a circular pattern. Massage very lightly for five minutes. Close your eyes or lower your gaze and be aware of how it feels. If you feel this point is extremely sensitive ease the pressure, and if it feels uncomfortable omit this point altogether. Keep breathing, as it is important not to neglect your breath.

Bai hui or 'hundred convergences' is located at the crown of the head, at the midway point of the line joining both apexes of the ears. This point is sensitive and energetically very alive and corresponds to the crown chakra. Bai hui calms your spirit and mind. It can alleviate anxiety, mental restlessness (which in traditional Chinese medicine is called *shen* or 'mind') and disturbances such as depression.

Place your thumbs at the apexes of your ears and allow your middle fingers to join at the top of your head. Allow yourself to feel where the bai hui acupoint is and place your middle finger on it. Apply very light pressure on the point, and if it feels as though it's too much then gently rest your finger there. Bring your attention to the point and hold this position for at least two to three minutes or longer if you can. Follow the rhythm of your breath and keep your mind focused on this point.

An mian or 'peaceful sleep' is located in the depression just behind the ears at the base of the skull. As the name indicates it is very good for insomnia, disrupted or agitated sleep through excessive dreaming (vivid or intense dreams that are not peaceful) and nightmares.

Place the tips of your index and middle fingers or thumbs on the an mian on both sides of your head. Massage in a circular motion for around five minutes. You should feel a deep sense of relaxation. Once again, follow the rhythm of your breath.

Special note: the head massage ritual is best performed at the end of the day or just before you go to bed, as it will help you to shake off any tension and promote relaxation for a peaceful sleep. When you grieve and experience great emotional trauma it creates blockages in the energy pathways or energy channels, which creates tension that often gets trapped in the upper part of your body and especially your head. This build up of tension manifests itself in many physical ailments such as insomnia, headaches, nightmares and mental restlessness.

You deserve to feel

whole again.

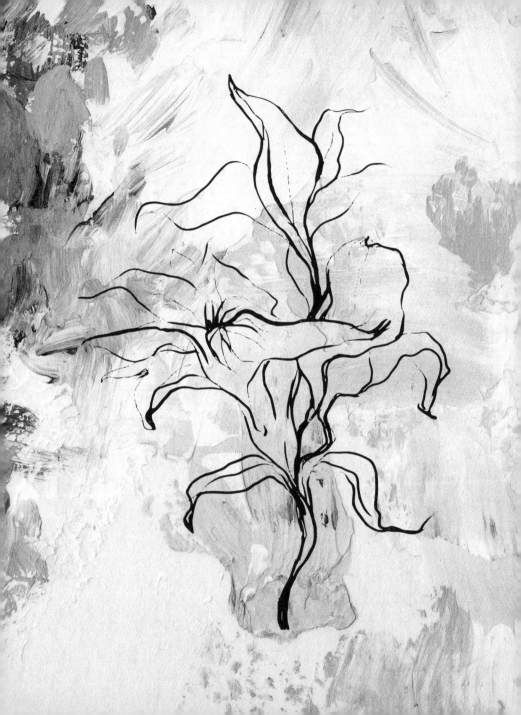

11

Spirit rituals
invisible allies

Spirit can mean different things to each one of us. Whether you look at spirit from a religious perspective or from a non-denominational point of view you know that spirit is infinite, invisible and immortal. Spirit lives both outside of and within you and flows through you. You can feel its presence at various times in your life or sense it around you in the stars and in gentle breezes and the trees. When you create the space to be fully present through rituals the manifestation of spirit becomes more apparent, and its guidance can help you on your journey of grief and healing.

1 *Herbal incense ritual*

The herbal incense ritual is a powerful tool on your healing journey, and I invite you to explore its magic with both wonder and an open heart. It will remove negative and stagnant energy from any space so you can be fully present and feel more grounded.

The burning of incense during rituals and ceremonies brings something magical to the whole experience; it goes back to ancient civilisations and is still being used in various cultures across the globe. The fragrant smoke is believed to have distinct divine powers and is experienced deep within the soul.

The fragrance that is released when incense is burned stimulates the senses, then in turn the mind is fully engaged and present in the here and now. The fragrance has both a relaxing and meditative effect on your mind and body, slowing you down and providing a moment to reconnect with yourself and the outside world.

Making a herbal incense for rituals is in itself immensely therapeutic. It requires blending together the intention of healing, plant energy, inner and outer energy and healing intuition to create magic and mystery.

This ancient practice must be used with the highest respect and with only the purest intention. Consciously transfer your intention and healing energy into your hands while choosing, mixing and crushing the herbs to bring intense peace and a wealth of wisdom to the whole process.

It is important for any preparation of this nature that you dedicate a space and use utensils unique for this purpose and treat them with great respect. Energetically cleanse yourself, the utensils and the space before every preparation to remove any negative energy.

You will need one or two wooden or clay bowls for mixing the herbs, a wooden spoon, a Mason jar to store the incense mix and a mortar and pestle to grind the herbs. I prefer using a mortar and pestle over an electric

grinder as the energy you create while grinding the ingredients goes into your blend. I also like to say a healing intention as I work with the herbs.

In the mortar, crush together:

- ¼ cup dried white sage (sage cleanses and balances energy)
- ¼ cup dried sweet grass (sweet grass calls upon spirit guides and ancient wisdom)
- 1 tablespoon palo santo wood chips (palo santo removes negative energy)

Use herbs that are locally available in your community. If you can't source the herbs listed then rosemary, pine sawdust, cedar or lemon balm can be used instead.

Take a moment to ground yourself and take a few breaths while you set your intention. As you prepare the incense, focus your mind and think of your intention, and thank the plant energy you are working with and Mother Earth for offering you these powerful healing plants. As you mix and crush the herbs together, visualise the healing properties of each herb. Call upon them to remove any negative energy that may have accumulated into your home or work space. Store the herbal incense in an airtight Mason jar.

Any time you feel disconnected from spirit because the energy within your home feels heavy, use the herbal incense mix to remove the stagnant energy. You can use this mix in the smoke and fire ritual in this chapter or the following quick method to cleanse your space and feel more connected to spirit.

Light a charcoal using an incense tong and place it in a stone bowl filled with sand. As you sprinkle a pinch of the incense mix over the charcoal repeat the following:

May the smoke cleanse this space. May I feel the gentle presence and guidance of spirit.

⦿ *Herbal love incense recipe*

To make the herbal love incense you will need:

- 4 tablespoons dried rose petals
- 4 tablespoons dried lavender
- 1 tablespoon fennel seeds (stability and security)
- 2 star anise (trust)
- 5 drops rose essential oil (love and transformation)
- 3 drops lavender essential oil (connection and cleansing)

The essential oils in this recipe will enhance the healing and purifying properties of the herbs.

Before you begin, connect with each herb and feel or sense the energy of the herbs through touch and smell. Take a few cleansing breaths to focus your mind and bring you to the here and now, and thank the plant energy you are going to work with and the beautiful generosity of Mother Earth for offering you these wonderful healing herbs.

Combine the first four ingredients in a mixing bowl. Transfer the herbs to a mortar and crush them with a pestle, all the time keeping your focus on your intention and feeling and sensing the energy of each herb. When you are ready, transfer the herbs back to the mixing bowl and add the essential oils, using a wooden spoon to mix everything well together.

You need to charge the herbal incense before using, and there are several ways you can do this. Pick the method that speaks to you the most or be guided by your intuition.

The earth and cosmic energy method: take a few cleansing breaths to ground yourself and focus your mind. Connect with the earth energy below and the cosmic energy above, visualising both energies being combined into one at the centre of your heart space. When you are ready, place both of your hands with the palms facing down over the mixing bowl containing the herbal mixture. Soften your hands and fingers; your shoulders and all the way down to your hands and fingertips should not hold any tension. Visualise the energy travelling from your heart space to your shoulders and down to your hands and charging the incense.

The crystal method: arrange rose quartz and clear quartz in a circle around the jar of incense. Let it charge for a good 24 hours.

The moon method: if you love working with the energy of the moon, this method is for you. Wait for the next full moon to make the herbal incense then place the jar on the windowsill, leaving it overnight to allow the full moon to supercharge it.

The herbal love incense can be used in two different ways: you can burn it using charcoal or you can burn it with a soya candle in a glass jar. To do the latter you will need to grind the ingredients into a fine powder, which can be done by grinding just a small amount at a time.

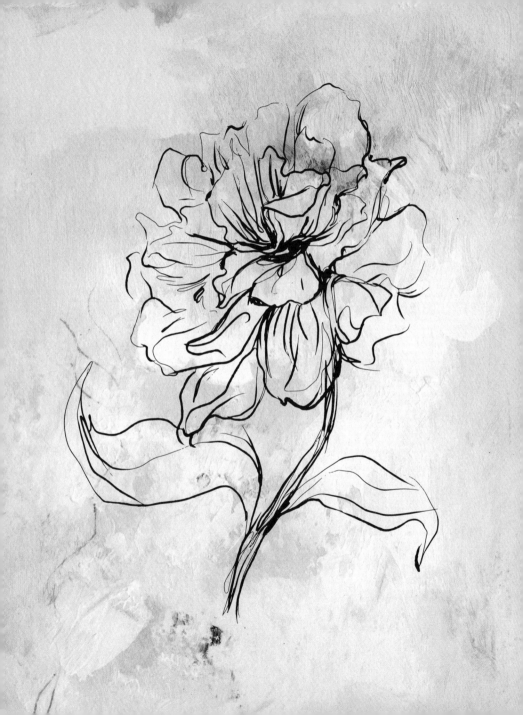

⦿ *Smoke and fire ritual*

For the smoke and fire ritual you will need the herbal incense mix above to remove negative energy, a stone bowl filled with sand, incense tongs and a charcoal tablet.

Take a moment to bring yourself into the here and now and be grounded. Hold the charcoal tablet on one end with the incense tongs and light the other end. Once lit, place the hot charcoal in the stone bowl.

Take a few cleansing breaths and bring forth your intention and desire to cleanse the space. Sprinkle a pinch of the herbal love incense onto the hot charcoal.

You may wish to repeat the following:

Smoke and fire: cleanse this space.
May only positive energy remain.

Continue to sprinkle pinches of the incense onto the hot charcoal, which should continue to burn for around 15 minutes.

When you are ready to close this ritual, thank the plant energy for its assistance.

Ⅳ *Love lives on ritual*

For the love lives on ritual, place a candle in your sacred space or somewhere in your home such as your living room. Set your intention and sprinkle the candle with a pinch or two of the fine powder from the herbal love incense.

Light the candle, and as you do so you may wish to recite a love poem or play your loved one's or your own favourite song. You may also want to sit in silence and remember your loved one that way. The choice is entirely yours, but whatever you do you are acknowledging that despite the loss love never dies, that love lives on.

You can use the candle several times, and each time before lighting the candle sprinkle a little more of the herbal incense on the candle.

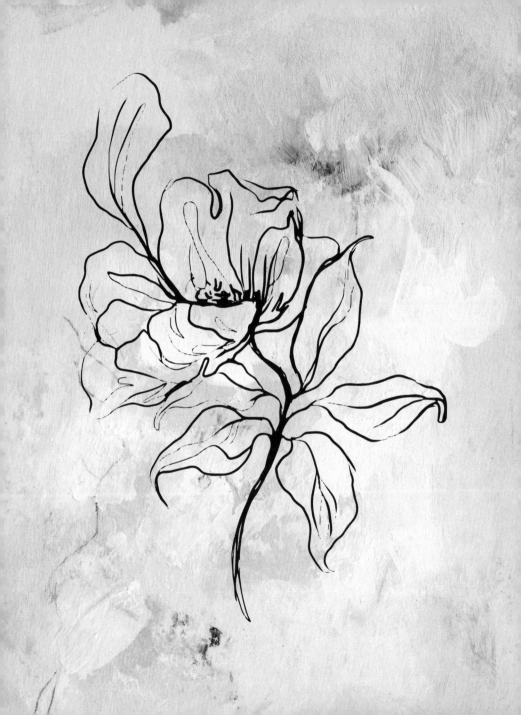

12

Rituals using the five elements

earth, water, fire, air and space

Reading Tenzin Wangyal Rinpoche's book *The True Source of Healing* was a pivotal point in my continued search for healing, which began with finding the balance within myself. Reconnecting with nature is a simple and wonderful way to find balance, inner peace and healing, and every small shift that occurs within you brings you one step closer to feeling grounded and living a more rewarding life. In this chapter I share five simple nature rituals using the five elements of earth, water, fire, air and space.

● *Earth ritual*

If you have been feeling disconnected, ungrounded and restless it is a call to reconnect with the earth. When you are grounded your thoughts will be less foggy and you can respond to your emotions with greater clarity.

A simple ritual to help you feel more grounded and less disconnected is to be barefoot outside in nature, as through your bare feet you connect with the energy of the earth. If you have one, your back garden will suffice. Find a quiet spot and kick off your shoes. Stand tall and imagine your feet spreading roots deep into the earth. Breathe and feel the subtle energy of the earth.

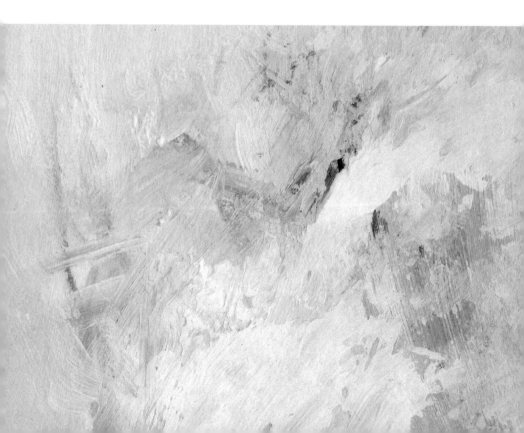

⓫ *Water ritual*

The fluidity of water invites you to flow with ease when you are faced with challenges. Water invites the flow of energy:

> *I will be water. I will flow effortlessly through the land. I will nourish the soil I touch. I will bring life in every shape and form where life didn't exist before, and maybe eventually I will find my healing.*

If you cannot find inner joy, are experiencing difficulties in your relationships with family and friends or you do not feel comfortable in your own skin like something is not quite right, this is a call to connect with the soothing and comforting energy of water.

In the shower or in the bath, make a conscious effort to connect with the water. If you can, go for a swim in a lake or in the sea; any body of water will do. Feel the water's fluidity and gentle reassuring touch and its comforting energy on your skin. Close your eyes and stay in the water for as long as you need to.

⑪ *Fire ritual*

Fire is all about the joy of life and boundless creativity. The fire ritual is perfect when you are feeling unsatisfied with life, are unhappy in your relationships with others or feel your creativity is not flowing with ease.

Make a fire or light a candle and watch the flames as they dance with vitality. Take a moment to feel the warmth of the fire as you soak it all up. Breathe deeply in and out a few times. In the summer months when the sun is shining, sit comfortably in a sunny spot, close your eyes and feel the warmth of the sun on your skin. Take a deep breath and connect with your inner fire, your inner joy and inner vitality.

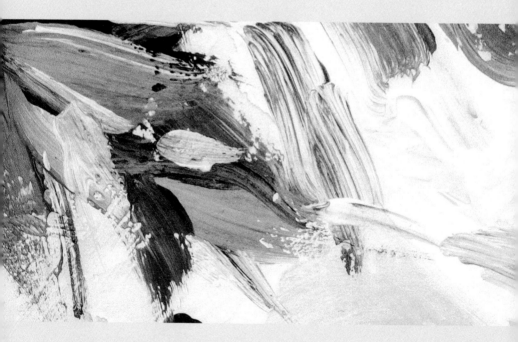

THE ART OF GRIEVING

Ⅳ *Air ritual*

Air is freedom. When you are in need of a fresh perspective on a particular situation or of shifting negative emotions into positive ones, or you simply feel stuck in a mundane routine the air ritual is a perfect invitation.

Find a quiet spot in nature such as the beach or a meadow or hilltop, anywhere you can feel the breeze. Make yourself comfortable either standing or sitting and close your eyes. Feel the delicate touch of the breeze on your face, arms and legs and feel your own inner flexibility. Imagine yourself moving with ease and freedom through the challenges you are facing.

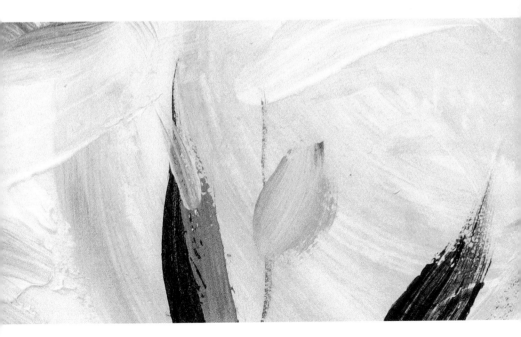

Ⓥ *Space ritual*

Space reminds you to keep your heart open without judgement of yourself or others. It is a gentle prompt to connect with your inner spaciousness. When you are feeling overwhelmed and weighted down, this ritual can help you approach challenges with an open heart and allow you to access your inner vastness with renewed energy and new resources to deal with difficult situations as well as tough emotions.

Choose a quiet, open and safe space in nature. If you live in the city and have access to a balcony or rooftop, that will do. Take a moment to deeply breathe in the beauty of your surroundings. Take a few cleansing breaths, slowly inhaling and exhaling. As you exhale, release all the tension in your body. When you are ready, soften your gaze a little and observe the sky above you, how vast it is. You are as vast as the sky; you are limitless; your heart has no boundaries, judgement or prejudice. Feel the openness of the sky and connect with your inner spaciousness. What you see above is a reflection of your inner space.

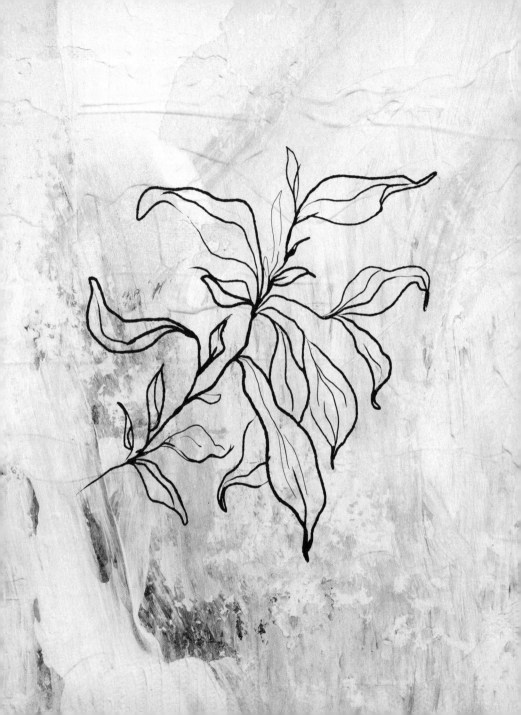

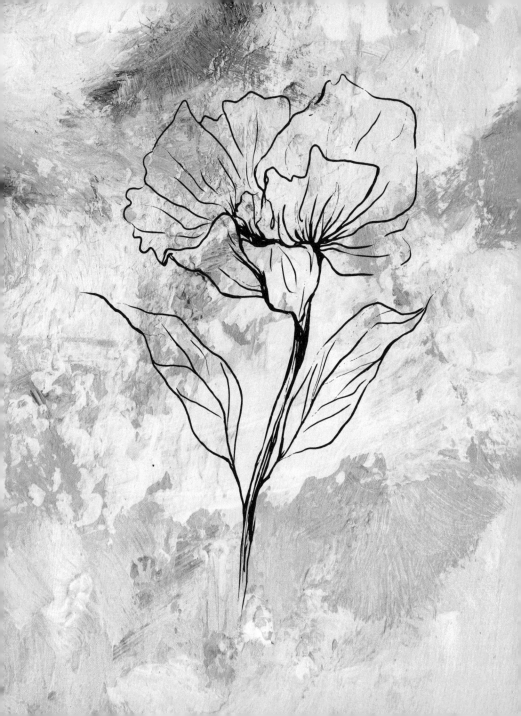

13

The healing power of words

creating flow

You use words every day to express what you need, want and feel. Words are powerful, and when you use them wisely you can make positive changes within as well as around you. I invite you to explore the healing power of words through the simple rituals outlined in this chapter.

Words are as soothing as a spoonful of honey to the wounded heart:

> *When I write I flow: I take shelter from the chaos; I listen to my soul's silent songs. My memories, my thoughts, my deepest emotions, my prayers and my dreams melt on crisp paper, revealing the secret wisdom held within. Healing words here and there are captured within the pages of my journal. There is indeed beauty in healing.*

Notes on grief ritual

This ritual is an invitation to capture your sorrow through words in the form of journaling and doodling. It provides a time for self-reflection, introspection without judgement and making room for self-healing. Through journaling your grief your awareness of the world around you and how you choose to respond to life experiences increases. Over time, the practice will create a shift in your consciousness and you will begin to make changes where changes are needed. As you keep filling the pages of your journal with notes on grief you will see the progress you have made along your healing journey.

You do not need to be a writer, write brilliantly or be grammatically correct; journaling is simply about capturing your grief, your thoughts and your hopes and dreams on paper. There is no right or wrong way to journal: as with your grief, your journal is unique and personal. When words are not enough or are difficult to record on paper, draw, scribble or use collage. You can take photographs and insert them in your journal or use paint or coloured ink to add vibrancy to the pages. Treat your journal as an extension of your spiritual self: your journal is sacred and holds the key to unlocking the beauty of your soul.

Make a date to write in your journal. Grab a cup of your favourite hot drink or beverage. Sit comfortably in your sacred space, take a deep breath and slowly close your eyes. Allow your intuition to guide you: what do you want to capture within the pages of your journal? Perhaps you want to document your emotions or thoughts from a recent event or today is an anniversary, a special day, a breakthrough in your journey so far. When you are ready, open your eyes and write.

If you feel compelled to fashion a unique journal, try the following creative activity that uses a plain A4 or A5 notebook, preferably with recycled paper,

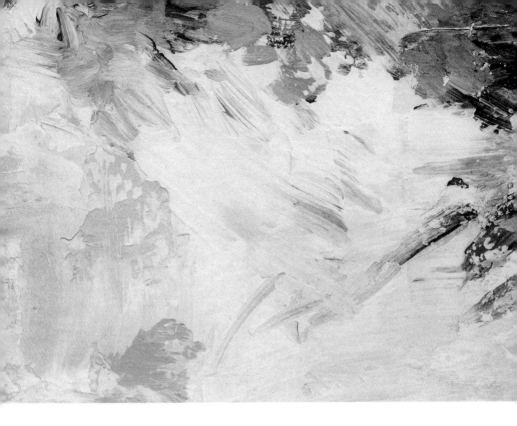

and mixed media for embellishment. You can use a variety of techniques to beautify the pages of your journal as well as the cover. For example, collage is not only eye-catching but brings texture and colour to otherwise plain pages. Cut pictures out of old magazines or draw your own straight into your journal. Another technique for adding colour to the pages is to spray ink onto them. If you use this technique, make sure the thickness of the paper can take it otherwise you will end up with wrinkled paper, and dilute some acrylic paint or ink in water so it doesn't clog in a spray bottle and lightly spray the pages. Use several colours for effect. Have fun and allow your creativity to flow.

❶ A letter to grief ritual

The letter to grief ritual can help you in your mourning process as it will allow you to express the sorrow you feel on the inside. You can perform this ritual once a week or once a month, whatever feels best for you.

Sit comfortably in your sacred space or in a quiet spot where you will be undisturbed. Take a few cleansing breaths and relax – there is no rush – and write your letter. Here is an example of a letter to grief:

> *Grief my dear old friend, here we are again on this grim day.*
> *I am not afraid; I can face your darkness and tight grip. I know this now:*
> *light always follows darkness and darkness always follows light.*
> *This is the nature of things. This is yin and yang; this is how life flows,*
> *the constant death and rebirth. So here I am: vulnerable but strong,*
> *lost but courageous. I trust from the depth of my soul that*
> *I will find my healing and my light over and over again. The tight*
> *grip you hold on me will not last. I am well. I am healing every day.*

When you are ready to complete this ritual, close your journal and take a deep breath in and out as you place your left hand on your heart space. Acknowledge this moment as a gift and a step forward on your healing journey. Every time you write a letter to grief you are allowing yourself to mourn and at the same time heal your broken heart.

⏸ *Poetry ritual*

Poetry, a word that is derived from the Greek word *poieo* meaning 'I create', is one of the most ancient forms of art. It was often used as a form of storytelling: through effective imagery, ideas and emotions were shared with a wide audience.

Poems have the ability to rearrange emotions and present them in a flow of words that is peaceful and soothing to your heart and soul. When you explore poetry the words awaken your empathy, love and compassion and can become a powerful healing tool. They bring peace to your mind, then eventually your body follows this cue and starts to relax. This internal shift can momentarily reduce stress in your body, a short break from stress that can be therapeutic.

Choose your favourite poem. Take a moment away from the chaos of life and sit comfortably in your sacred space. Read the poem out loud, feeling the vibration of the words. You can also capture a beautiful poem in your journal or compose your own poem on grief, healing, death, life and love. Allow your inner poet to surface. Here is an example:

> *Tears like spring rain*
> *Please wash away my pain and deep sorrow*
> *Like the sun softly kisses the earth at dawn*
> *Let me feel the warm rays of love again deep within my wounded soul.*

⦿ *Affirmation ritual*

Words carry vibrations and powerful energy both positive and negative. They can dictate your mindset and influence your behaviour, and can uplift your spirit or take you deeper into a downward spiral. It is not only words someone else says to you, but those words that float continuously in your mind throughout the day that you have uttered to yourself both consciously and subconsciously. Take a moment to reflect on which words occupy your mind. If your mind is filled with negative self-talk, this affirmation ritual will help you to shift your mindset.

An affirmation is a sentence or phrase composed of positive words you can repeat out loud or silently on a regular basis or whenever you need a helping hand to guide you through a particularly tough time. When you are facing the world alone, barely surviving and your vulnerability is suddenly exposed, it is tough to be decisive and confident. The affirmation ritual is simply an infusion of genuine words that can uplift your mood and boost your self-confidence, self-esteem and trust. Infusing your world with positive words helps you to achieve your life goals with ease and less self-doubt, encouraging you to leave behind any negative thoughts that may be holding you back.

When you repeat an affirmation you are making a conscious effort and commitment to shift the way you think about yourself and the world around you. Positive affirmation can help to shake off negative thoughts that may have been haunting your mind since your devastating loss. Furthermore, a positive affirmation can help you tap into your innate wisdom and inner power.

When you first start a positive affirmation ritual you may feel some resistance, as for any great change to occur discomfort is necessary. This resistance is asking you to raise the bar higher, to dig deeper and create the change you want to achieve. It takes commitment and repetition to create meaningful changes.

I encourage you to write an affirmation that has special meaning for you. If you find it difficult to write your own, use the following affirmation in your ritual:

I am healing. Each day I find new courage and new strength to move forward. I am worthy of love. I am at peace.

Your sacred space is the perfect spot to conduct this ritual. Set your intention as you light a candle and take a few deep, cleansing breaths. Repeat your affirmation as many times as you need or until you feel a shift within you.

Close the ritual by releasing a positive word or words into the universe.

Tip: commit to at least one week of daily positive affirmation, and capture your experience of practising this ritual in your journal so you can note what changes have occurred in your mindset and behaviour.

As the key to positive affirmation is repetition and you need to repeat the affirmation several times for it to start working its magic, you may wish to include a meditation bead in your practice. A meditation bead is a wonderful tool for focusing your mind that is very similar to a prayer bead; over time your mind will instinctively make the connection between a positive mindset and the meditation bead. At moments when sorrow comes crashing down on you like a huge wave, simply holding the meditation bead can bring peace and gentle support.

If you would like to make a meditation bead to accompany your daily affirmation then try this fun creative activity. You can buy a meditation or prayer bead, but making your own will give you the opportunity to create something that is unique and personal and in which you can immerse sacred beauty.

You can add beads, crystals and charms that hold special meaning for you. These can be crystal beads that hold energetic power, a pendant that has great significance to you and sea shells, which are known for their healing and balancing energy. The material and how you wish to create the meditation bead is entirely your choice. You can use a three by three pattern and make it as long or as short as you wish. The most important aspect of this activity is the creating part and making something that holds meaning and purpose for you. Regardless of the pattern you use or the material you choose, the meditation bead is a personal and powerful ally you can use every day for as long as you need.

You will need for nine beads (crystals beads such as amethyst, clear quartz or rose quartz work well), six small spacers, four larger spacers, wax cord and two differently sized pendants. Attach one end of the cord to the bigger pendant with a knot, then add one big spacer and string three beads with a small spacer in between each one. Between each section of three beads add a bigger spacer. To finish, add a bigger spacer before securing the smaller pendant at the end.

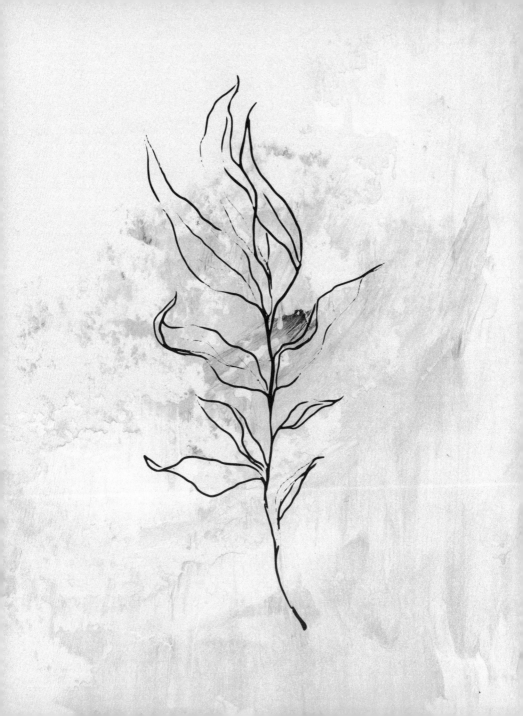

14

Stone medicine: a crystal invitation

healing gems of the earth

Working with crystals is a natural and gentle approach to holistic healing that dates back to ancient times, with all of its wisdom meticulously recorded in scriptures. Crystals are not only beautiful, but they hold magical and powerful healing properties. Even if you do not believe in magic, there is something quite special about crystals: they have a certain subtle, quiet and peaceful energy.

The healing qualities of crystals can be drawn upon at any time on your healing journey to bring balance to your energy field and clarity to your mind, and a general sense of well-being and inner peace.

Crystals for healing grief

Below is a list of some of the crystals you might like to explore.

- **Quartz:** clear or white in colour, quartz can channel any energy and is very good for healing and balancing your emotions. It can help to focus your mind as well as remove any negative energy.

- **Citrine:** a variety of quartz that can be yellow, golden or lemon in colour. Citrine can help to boost self-esteem and get rid of emotional toxins such as anger and is a beautiful crystal to balance yin and yang.

- **Jade:** this crystal comes in a wide range of colours such as green, orange, brown, blue, lavender, red, grey, black, cream and white. It can help with grounding and enhances confidence, as well as promoting emotional balance. It is an excellent crystal for inner and outer peace and for wisdom.

- **Unakite:** this very interesting stone is a mixture of quartz, feldspar and epidote that can help with accepting past experiences and moving forward in life from a place of love.

- **Rose quartz:** this crystal, which has a very soft pink appearance and a very calming effect, can help with releasing grief, stress, anger, fear, guilt and emotional wounds. It enhances forgiveness and is an excellent crystal for love.

- **Peridot:** this green stone can also be found in red, yellow and brown. Peridot can clear emotional blockages and allows a fresh outlook on life. It is an amazing crystal for clearing stress, anger and depression.

Additional crystals for healing grief

- **Amethyst:** a wonderful, usually purple crystal for releasing negative energy such as guilt, rage and sorrow that is often worn as a piece of jewellery to bring a sense of calm to the wearer. If you have been finding it difficult to fall asleep or are experiencing restless nights and nightmares, place an amethyst crystal under your pillow or place it on your bedside cabinet as it can help soothe your grief.

- **Moonstone:** this crystal helps to release energy blocks, encourages compassion and calms and balances emotions. It is a perfect ally if you are feeling numb and disconnected, especially in the early stages of grief. You can find moonstone in various colours, the most common ones being cream, white and rainbow.

- **Obsidian:** a powerful crystal that may be too strong to use in the very early stages of grief, although it is excellent for grounding. Obsidian comes in many hues including black, brown and mahogany.

- **Apache tears:** well-known for healing grief, Apache tears are a version of obsidian that come in black or brown that are good for the early stages of grief. They encourage emotional balance and forgiveness and soothe painful emotions, and can remove negativity.

- **Onyx:** another wonderful crystal for relieving deep sorrow that can help when you need to take charge of situations and life challenges. Onyx, a multicoloured crystal with black, brown, red, orange, white, grey and blue tones, can balance yin and yang energy.

Working with crystals

Choosing a crystal is a very personal matter: some may resonate with you and you may be immediately attracted to them, while others may give you a different vibe, a certain reluctance to want to touch or hold them. However, every crystal – even the ones you may not feel attracted to – has something to offer. Take your time when choosing a crystal or crystals: touch, feel and listen and trust your intuition. Touch is a good way to know if a crystal is the right one for you. Close your eyes and listen deeply with your heart: is this the right crystal for you?

Before you start working with crystals it is best to cleanse them; they need regular cleansing and should be well looked after. These wonderful stones tend to absorb energy from their environment, other people and yourself, and dust can affect their healing properties. If your crystals look dusty you can use a soft paint brush or make-up brush to loosen and remove the dust from their surfaces.

To cleanse your crystals you can smudge them with white sage, palo santo or incense and allow the smoke to waft over them. You can also place the crystals in natural sunlight, but be careful not to leave clear quartz in direct sunlight as it can become a fire hazard. Some crystals may lose their vibrant colour in direct sunlight. If you prefer working with the gentle energy of the moon, place your crystals under moonlight and especially on a new moon or full moon depending on what your intention is. Choose a new moon if you are using the crystals for healing or a full moon if you would like to enhance the crystals' properties.

THE ART OF GRIEVING

❶ *Crystal ritual*

When your crystal has been cleansed, sit quietly in your sacred space and hold the crystal in the palm of your hands. Close your eyes and take a few cleansing breaths, releasing any tension in your body as you exhale. Take a couple of deep breaths and focus your mind on your crystal, connecting with it not only in your mind but also in your heart. Think of the crystal's healing properties as you ask yourself these questions. What do you need from the crystal? What is your deepest intention? Feel, sense or visualise the colour of the crystal surrounding you like a shield with its protective and healing energy. Allow yourself five to 10 minutes to explore and connect with the crystal.

When you are ready, open your eyes and place your crystal on your altar. Your crystal is now tuned in to you.

When you feel in need of extra support, hold your crystal in your hand. Take a few deep breaths, close your eyes and connect with the crystal and visualise, feel or sense its protective shield surrounding you. Take a moment; there is no rush. Once you feel calmer, your heart feels more at peace and you feel rested, slowly open your eyes.

ⅠⅠ *Crystal bundles*

If you love the therapeutic energy of crystals you can create a crystal bundle for healing. Choose three tumbled crystals or mini-sized crystals from the list above or any other crystals that hold special meaning for you. Use a piece of cord or ribbon to securely tie the crystals within a piece of colourful fabric or contain them within a small pouch.

This small bundle is easy to carry with you in your pocket or your purse and will give you extra support whenever you are facing challenges.

THE ART OF GRIEVING

◉ *Magic three crystals ritual*

There are three particular crystals that soothe and balance the mind, heart and soul.

Amethyst is the healing stone of choice for grief as it reduces sorrow and helps to release negative energy such as guilt, self-blame, anger and rage. It also removes emotional blockages and will soothe your heart. **Rose quartz** is a beautiful gentle stone that is perfect for healing deep sorrow as it opens and purifies your heart. It can soothe anger by promoting love, in particular self-love, and brings balance and inner peace. **Clear quartz** is a powerful healing crystal that promotes clarity of mind and amplifies the energy of the other two crystals.

Place one each of these crystals in a triangular shape in your sacred space or in any room in which you spend the majority of your day or even on your desk at work. You can easily move them around your home, for example into your bedroom, living room or study. If you're finding it difficult to fall asleep, place them on your bedside cabinet. Take a few deep breaths and visualise the crystals' protective healing energy infusing your space and casting a protective healing shield around you.

Take care of your crystals by cleansing them regularly.

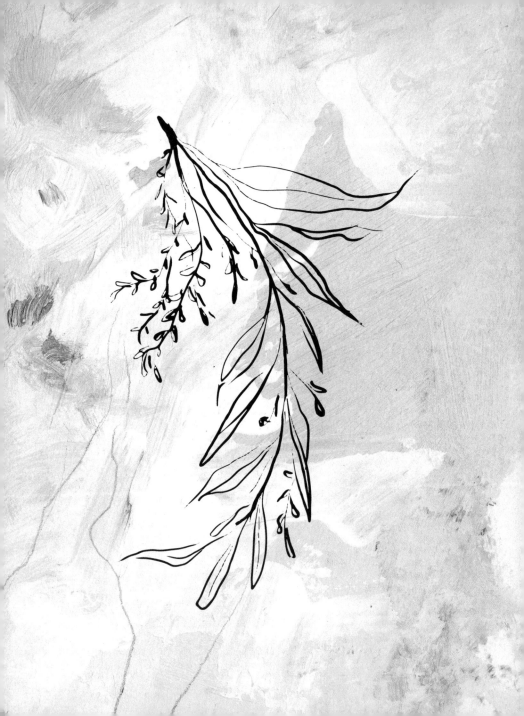

15

Energy rituals
balance and flow

We are all made of energy, the countless electrical impulses and chemical reactions that occur in our bodies. When your body is in balance energy flows uninterrupted to nourish the organs and every cell, sustaining life. An abundance of energy is particularly essential for maintaining good health.

Stress and emotional trauma have an adverse effect on your body's energy. The emotional shock of a loss and any unresolved grief that follows can linger for a very long time and have a harmful effect on your general health and well-being if it is not addressed properly. Eventually it will start to affect your ability to connect with others and can instigate mood swings as well as depression.

Stress can cause an obstruction in the free flow of energy that can further worsen emotional and physical issues. Your body is a vessel that is constantly moving internally and constantly adjusting to inside and outside forces. This quote by Japanese master Do Hyun Choe encapsulates this essence: 'Stillness is what creates love. Movement is what creates life. To be still yet still moving, that is everything.' Tai chi and qi gong were developed in China to cultivate energy in order to promote health and well-being.

❶ *Breath ritual*

We often go about our day paying little or no attention to our breath. In yoga the breath is referred to as *prana*, meaning 'life force'. In other disciplines such as qi gong the breath is referred to as *qi* (pronounced 'chee'). All these ancient arts teach us how to harvest the most out of our breath.

The breath is an invisible vital force that sustains life and can help you heal your physical body. When you learn to use your breath correctly you can feel revitalised or calmer if you experience a bout of anxiety or stress. The breath does not require any special equipment; it only requires your attention, curiosity and commitment to explore its possibilities.

THE ART OF GRIEVING

The breath ritual can be a perfect morning ritual before starting your day or whenever you feel anxious or overwhelmed by strong emotions.

Sit or stand with your spine straight, your shoulders down and your chest open and slowly close your eyes to help focus your attention. Bring your awareness to your breath, feeling the air enter your nostrils and move downwards to your lungs. Feel your lungs expand as you breathe in and deflate as you breathe out.

Take a deep breath through your nose, using the entire capacity of your lungs, and exhale fully in a long breath that allows your lungs to gently deflate. When you are ready, take another deep breath followed by another long exhale. Follow the rhythm of your breath; it should never be forced and should always feel natural.

Repeat the inhale and exhale nine times, then bring your attention back to your surroundings and slowly open your eyes. You should now feel calm and energised at the same time.

As you continue to practise with the breath you'll notice the subtle space between the in breath and the out breath and the out breath and the in breath, almost as if you are suspended in time and space in complete stillness and there is no conscious effort from your body. This subtle, delicate space is where nothing is happening yet your body is being fully supported and nourished. It is a powerful reminder to slow down and to trust, and a surrendering to inner peace and deep healing.

❚❚ *Standing still ritual*

The practice of standing as still as a tree to gain inner peace and vitality is known as *zhan zhuang*. It dates back 4,000 years and has its roots in ancient China, with the first record of the practice being found in one of the oldest books of Chinese medicine, the *Nei Ching* by Huang Ti.

Energy known as qi flows through your entire body similar to blood in the vascular system. Its flow is constant and natural, like your breath or the beating of your heart. The Taoists, the very first alchemists, were fascinated by this life force as their primary goal was to preserve health and longevity. They developed a system to cultivate qi known as *qi gong*, with *qi* meaning 'life force' and *gong* meaning 'to cultivate'.

Taoists observe nature as a way of making sense of the human body. A tree looks very similar to the human body, with the legs/trunk, the feet/ roots and the head and arm/branches. Trees reach deep into the earth with their roots and their branches reach up towards the sky, the cosmos. A tree may look inactive and still but it is constantly gathering energy, and it is from this early observation that the practice of standing still like a tree emerged and it is part of classical qi gong.

Standing still in full awareness and intention helps to reboot your nervous system while at the same time deeply relaxing your body. When qi (energy) flows without obstruction it can increase the feeling of well-being. The practice may look simple to the onlooker, but when performed correctly its benefits can reach the deeper layers of your body. If you are experiencing grief, emotional trauma, stress and anxiety you should give the standing still ritual a try. If you are feeling run down and generally depleted, it can create enough space for your body's innate healing ability to emerge. Whenever your mind and body seem to be disconnected, this ritual can re-establish connection.

The best time is first thing in the morning and, if you can, you should be surrounded by trees, although indoors in a well-ventilated room will work just as well. The more you perform this ritual the quicker you will see the benefits. Make sure you are wearing comfortable clothes, and begin by doing a five minute ritual then gradually build up to 20 minutes.

You first need to do a warm up. Stand with your feet together, then bend your knees and lean over slightly so you can reach your knees with your fingers. From the waist up your body should be relaxed; avoid tension in your neck by gazing at a point a couple of metres in front of you. Place your hands on your knees and make 30 circles, first clockwise and then 30 circles anticlockwise.

Stand up straight with your feet shoulder width apart, your toes pointing forward and your knees unlocked. Allow your arms to hang loosely from your sides and your fingers to ever so slightly open and curve naturally. Visualise yourself being suspended by a string on the top of your head just like a puppet, completely letting go and allowing your body to soften. With each calm, easy breath, relax and sink further into the ground.

Stand in complete stillness for five minutes, giving your entire body a chance to unwind and your nervous system to readjust and make the switch to relaxation. Allow your gaze to gently drop to the ground somewhere in front of you. Lower your chin a little to release any tension that may have gathered at the back of your neck. Relax your jaw muscles and your shoulders and elbows. Continue to work on your entire body, including relaxing your hips and abdomen. Allow the bottom of your spine to unfold downwards. Keep inhaling and exhaling through your nose.

You may experience some resistance with this ritual, especially on your first attempt; frustration and boredom are common. If you experience these reactions it is a hint your body needs the practice. When resistance arises, remember you are an energy vessel with the ability to cultivate your energy and restore your health and well-being and ultimately enjoy a good life.

ⅠⅠⅠ *Five zang ritual*

In traditional Chinese medicine (TCM) there are five main organs that play an important part in keeping the body in balance, each of which is in turn associated with an emotion: the lungs are linked with grief; the heart with joy; the liver with anger; the kidneys with fear; and the spleen with worry. When the organs are referred to in TCM it indicates their energy.

To restore and maintain good health and well-being each of the five organs needs to be in harmony within itself and with the other organs. This is a simplified illustration of the five zangs working in harmony:

Slowly close your eyes and take a few cleansing breaths. Release any tension in your body as you exhale and relax a little further with each breath. Bring your attention to your heart, imagining it being in complete harmony within itself and everything externally. Take your time; there is no rush.

Visualise or sense this perfect harmony being sent to your spleen, which is now in harmony within itself and everything externally. Visualise your spleen conveying the harmony to your lungs, which are now in harmony within themselves and everything externally. Visualise your lungs sending this energy to your kidneys, which are now in harmony within themselves and everything externally. Visualise your kidneys continuing this process by sending the harmony to your liver, which is now in harmony within itself and everything externally.

To complete the circle, visualise your liver sending the flawless harmony back to your heart. Take a moment to visualise each organ being in perfect harmony within itself and in harmony with the other organs. As you continue to breathe, feel the inner peace as it gently moves throughout your body and visualise the peace spreading to every cell in your body.

When you are ready, bring your attention back to your surroundings and slowly open your eyes. Close this ritual with a grateful heart.

 *Qi flow ritual*

The qi flow ritual can be done whenever you feel the energy in your body has become stuck, which can be manifested by your feeling overly tired or easily distracted. The ritual can be revitalising as well as grounding and can bring calmness to a restless mind.

This ritual taps into the wisdom of TCM and the benefits of working with two very important meridians: the *ren mai* and the *du mai*. The Chinese word *mai* can be translated as 'meridian', 'channel' or 'vessel'. *Ren* has a deeper meaning, but for this ritual we will use its reference to nourishment of the life function. *Du* can be seen as being the leader who keeps a watchful eye over everything in order for the body to flourish.

Imagine a channel or meridian starting from your perineum area and running all the way up the front of your body and ending just in the depression below your lower lip. This is the ren mai or conception meridian. Next, imagine a channel starting from an area between your coccyx and anus that runs upwards along your spine all the way up to the crown of your head, continues towards your forehead and finishes at the junction of your gums and frenulum. Keep the path of the two meridians in mind.

Stand with your feet hip width apart and contract your anus and vagina or penis in order to keep the energy within your body. Soften your knees and relax your shoulders, then take a few deep breaths to relax any tension in your body. Place the tip of your tongue just behind your top teeth and touching your palate. The ren mai and the du mai are now connected and the energy circuit is complete.

Imagine the earth's energy coming up through your feet to join the energy circuit up your spine and heavenly energy from the cosmos coming in through your crown to also join the energy circuit. As you breathe, imagine this energy circulating back up and to the front and back again. It is a continuous flow of energy travelling through your body, energising and replenishing it. Keep visualising this flow of energy for a few minutes.

When you are ready to complete this ritual, slowly open your eyes and give thanks to the earth and cosmos energy for their constant support.

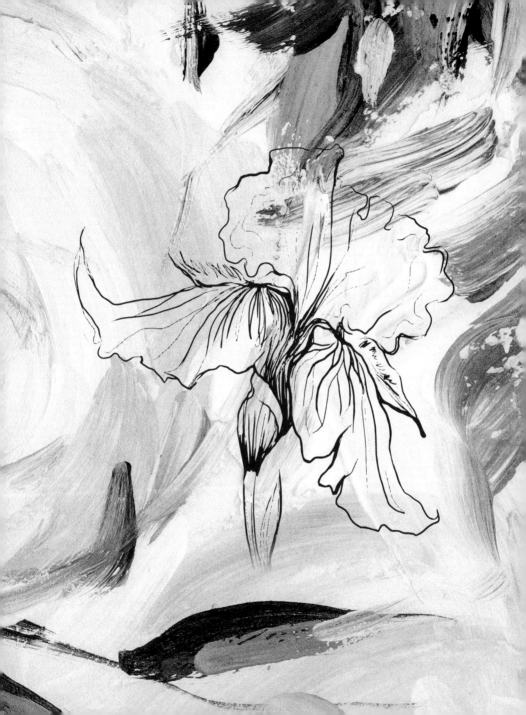

16

A mother's grief

love never ends

Mothers with empty arms, empty cradles and aching hearts: I see you. I want you to know that every life, no matter how brief or how small, matters.

You became a mother the very moment your womb holds life and your heart opens wide ready to welcome this new soul into your life and into this world. You fell in love with this tiny new life, the child you will never see growing up. Your souls connected; your hearts connected and love grew like wildfire through the landscape of your being. This is love in its purest form, so do not carry any guilt for loving so deeply.

All you can do after your overwhelming loss is hold the memory of your cherished baby with love in the most precious vessel you possess: your mother's heart. No one understands your heartache or the deep sorrow that keeps ripping you apart over and over again. Your world has collapsed yet your grief is silent and invisible.

I invite you here to take a deep breath, slow down, grieve and mourn your loss.

❶ *Womb ritual*

Often after a miscarriage you may feel disconnected from your womb or resentment towards it, along with anger, shame or even guilt. I once gave an abdominal massage to a young woman who had experienced a miscarriage several years previously. After the massage she told me this was the first time in years she had felt connected to her abdomen and especially her womb again. This is a common theme I hear over and over again. In traditional Chinese medicine the heart and the womb are connected through the *bao* vessel or *bao* channel, and any trauma in the womb can cause a blockage in the bao vessel. The communication link between the heart, which also happens to be the seat of the mind, is broken and the feeling of being disconnected with the womb arises.

Find a quiet space such as your sacred space. You can choose calming meditation music to play in the background if it helps you to relax. Sit comfortably on a chair or on the floor, take a few deep breaths and relax into your seat.

When you are ready, slowly close your eyes and bring your left hand onto your heart space and your right hand onto your womb space. Take nice easy breaths, allowing your abdomen to rise and fall with each inhale and exhale. Visualise a path unfolding between your heart and womb spaces and bring your attention to this path. With each breath, visualise energy flowing freely and easily from your heart space to your womb space. Stay there for a moment, and continue to visualise energy flowing with ease and abundance like a constant stream.

When you are ready to complete this ritual, bring both of your hands in a prayer pose in front of your heart space. Take a deep breath and slowly open your eyes.

To close this ritual, drink a cup of herbal infusion to warm your body.

ⓘ *Womb massage ritual*

This simple ritual will help you to connect to your womb space and abdomen and has therapeutic benefits that are more about reducing stress and promoting relaxation. You can make it a daily ritual after your bath or shower or just before bedtime.

Place a towel underneath you and get comfortable on a chair or on the floor. Pour a few drops of massage oil into your palms and rub the oil gently all over your abdomen (I love to blend 30 ml of almond oil with three drops each of rose and lavender essential oils). Start just below your belly button and rub clockwise in small circular movements all around your belly button using the soft tips of your index, middle and ring fingers to make the movements. As you massage your abdomen, pay attention to how your belly feels: is it tense, sensitive or cold? Apply as much pressure as you feel comfortable with.

Continue to massage and then gradually start to make the circle you have created around your belly button bigger until you have massaged your whole abdominal area including your womb space. Apply more massage oil if needed. Take the time to connect with your abdomen and womb; the massage should feel gentle and not rushed. Once you have completed the massage, place both of your hands on your abdomen. Take a few deep breaths and stay there for a moment. How does your belly feel: softer? Warmer?

To complete this ritual, cover yourself with a warm blanket and listen to some relaxation music or a guided meditation.

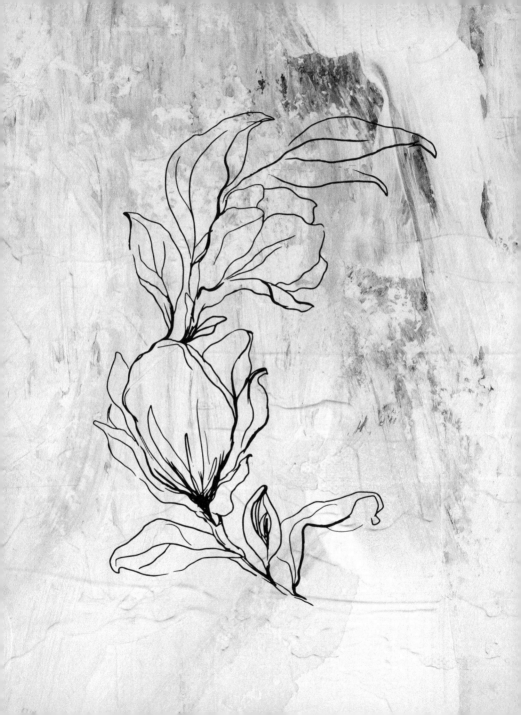

17

Collective grief rituals

coming together to ease deep sorrow

When the whole community is grieving and you feel lost in uncertainty, anxiety and emotional pain, dig deep into your ability to meet yourself with compassion. It is so easy to lose hope and faith when you are faced with immense grief. Keeping your grief hidden will only bring further suffering, so open up about your grief to others as you may be surprised to find you are not alone.

There are a few things you can do to ease collective grief within your community such as organising a collective grief circle ritual. Ask everyone who attends to bring something that for them represents hope and love and share their stories. If the collective grief concerns the death of someone in the community, shared stories about them can bring great comfort. You could create an altar with flowers and symbols that are important to you or light a candle in memory of the loss the community has suffered.

An important part of grieving is being witnessed and heard. After everyone has had a chance to share their stories you can close the circle with a collective prayer. You can use the following prayer I wrote, 'A Little Prayer for Dark Times', or a prayer of your choice that has a spiritual connection for your community:

May hope guide my every step

May faith keep me on the right path

May courage fill my broken heart

May strength fuel my spirit

May love give me shelter when the storm reaches my soul.

① *Memorial ritual*

You can organise a yearly memorial ritual in honour of the deceased. The memorial can take different shapes depending on what the deceased most loved. Host a sports day at the local community field or a bake and share day at your local church or in your own backyard. The list of things you can do is limitless and they can all bring so much comfort and joy.

Spend some time planning your event. Have a photograph of the deceased on an altar and write opening and closing speeches. Invite a spiritual leader to say a few words at the event if that seems appropriate. Make it a day full of joy wrapped in compassion.

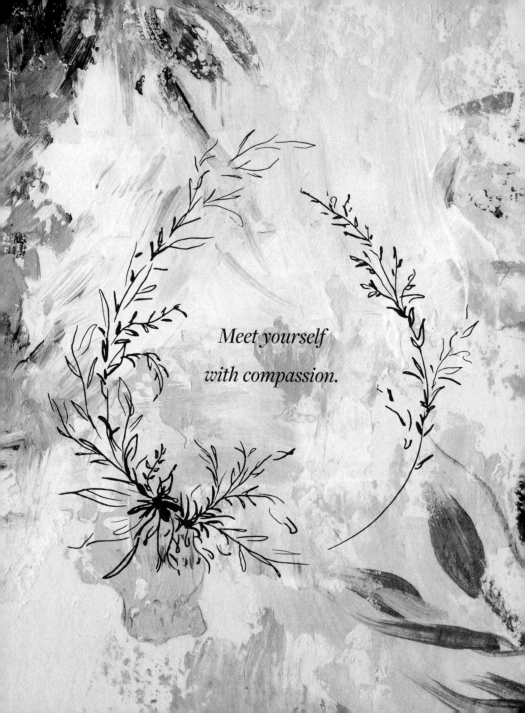

Meet yourself

with compassion.

18

New beginnings
embracing the future ahead

Despite having lost everything – from a joyous life to the innocence of love – don't allow yourself to fall into the bottomless pit of eternal pain. The path to wholeness is having the courage to be vulnerable and embracing the future with curiosity. Now is the time to forgive yourself and let go of self-blame, jealousy and anger and any other emotion that may be holding you back and dragging you down. Free yourself from the shackles of suffering and re-awaken your curiosity towards life and everything it has to offer. Every new day is an invitation to dive into the gift of life whether it is messy, beautiful or filled with mysteries. Open your heart to the new possibilities ahead of you as it is you and you only who holds the key to your future.

As you take the first steps on the path of new beginnings it is good to set yourself some short- and long-term goals. As with any large project, embracing the future or creating a new life requires careful planning, trust in the path ahead and a firm belief that anything is possible. You have the ability to turn things around and live a life filled with joy despite the pain of the past. The rituals described in this chapter can assist you as you make a fresh start.

❶ *Make a wish ritual*

An important part of healing is to still have hope and faith for the future. When I was going through a tough time a friend of mine gave me a wish bracelet that I wore every day; it never left my wrist. Every time I looked at the bracelet it reminded me of my wish and brought me comfort. Did my wish come true? Yes, it did. Did the bracelet hold special magic? I don't know, but I want to believe it had some magic. I think life is all about believing in possibilities even when they seem impossible. Regardless, one thing is for sure: every day it reminded me to take the steps necessary to make my wish come true.

To make a wish bracelet, thread a 25 cm cord through a small bead of your choice. As you tie the bracelet around your wrist, make a wish and silently repeat the following:

I wish . . . [state what you desire].
So it is from this day forward.

Wear the bracelet on your wrist to always remind you to keep your wish or hope alive.

▌ *Visualise the future ritual*

A fantastic tool to add to your rituals, visualisation is all about accessing the power of your mind so it can assist you in achieving your goals. Visualisation will have a calming effect on your mind and body, making your thoughts a lot clearer.

Your sacred space is the perfect place for this ritual. Take a few cleansing breaths and set your intention, then slowly close your eyes and visualise the future you would like to create. Perhaps you see yourself in a new home or job; perhaps you see yourself more at peace and settled in a fresh rhythm of life. Take your time.

As you see yourself in this new scenario, embrace the mood or emotion that arises. The emotions you feel can be strong, so receive yourself with compassion and love.

As you close this ritual, repeat the following silently:

> *I am ready to take the steps I need to create a future for me. I am strong and capable. My goal is within reach.*

● *Divine help ritual*

This ritual can be done when you need to make an important decision that will have a major impact on your future or you need to take the next step on your journey and it all feels a little scary.

Place a white candle on the altar in your sacred space. As you light the candle, ask for the guidance of God or the divine spirit then ask for the path ahead to be lit with pure light, with positive energy, and for all obstacles big and small to be removed.

When you are ready, close the ritual with a grateful heart. You can leave the candle burning if it is safe to do so or you can snuff it out.

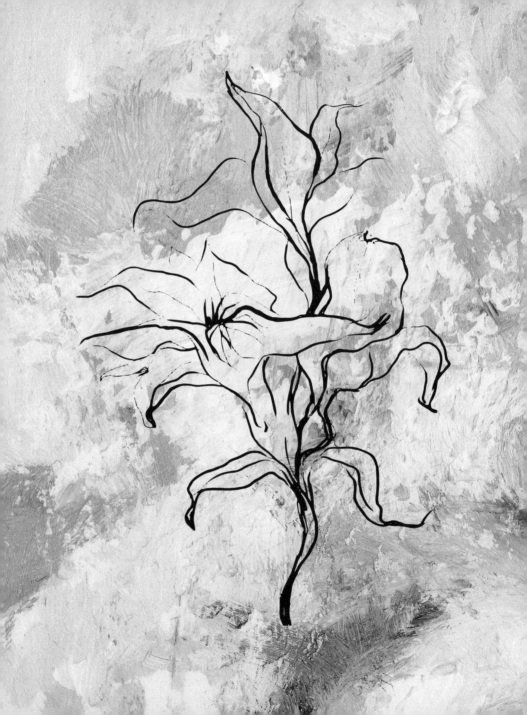

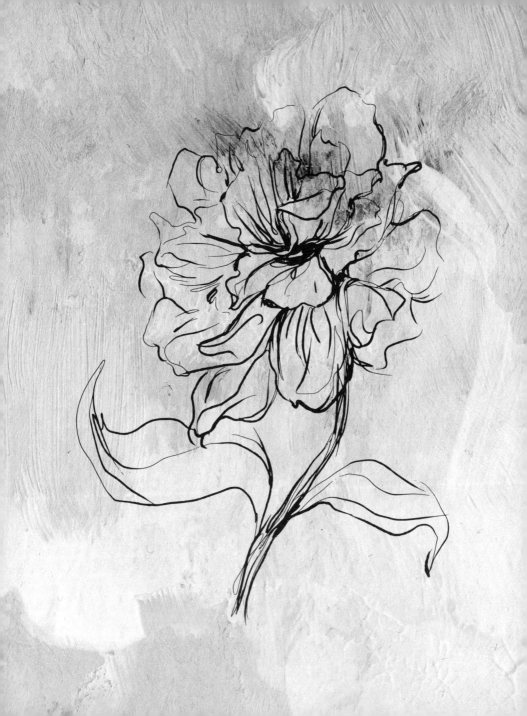

19

Ceremonies

to honour, to remember and to bless

A mourning ceremony is a self-care ritual that gives sorrow space to be transformed. To heal the fragmented pieces of your heart you must mourn and you must express your sorrow; by giving it a voice you can feel all of your emotions fully. Nothing goes unnoticed, because to heal your body and soul your emotions need to be taken care of with love and compassion.

Every culture has its own mourning tradition and rituals. The Aztecs, for example, used flowers to show departed souls their way back to earth and the Japanese have the memorial ceremony for unborn babies known as *mizuko kuyō*. All the mourning ceremonies worldwide share a few things in common: to remember, to acknowledge the presence of spirit and to give love and peace.

When you engage in a mourning ceremony you will gradually learn to live with the grief that is now a part of who you are. Above all, the beauty of ceremonies is that they bring a healing spark to your journey.

❶ *Ceremony for the departed soul*

Flowers are a symbol of the eternal cycle of life and death: they blossom in spring only to fade away in winter and disappear completely, then return again the following spring. It is a reminder that this life is only temporary but we do return again some day. The Aztec practice of using flowers to show departed souls their way back to earth was perhaps a very early recognition that despite the fact life is temporary the soul is eternal.

The colours of the flowers and the types of flowers chosen have great significance in mourning. White roses evoke innocence, reverence and purity while red roses evoke courage and love. White lilies are often chosen for funeral bouquets because lilies symbolise innocence and sympathy.

The act of lighting candles during ceremonies has great significance. In most cultures, candles and oil lamps are lit during ceremonies as a symbol of love, celebration, honouring and remembrance and of the triumph of light over darkness. The flame of a lit candle or oil lamp symbolises the light of the soul, a light that lives on in another form and is eternal.

You can choose a special place in nature for this ritual or your sacred space can provide the perfect spot; just make sure it's a place where you have privacy and can spend several minutes undisturbed in silence to honour the departed soul or souls.

Place a white candle or oil lamp next to your altar and lay a white flower beside the candle. Take a few cleansing breaths then light the candle or oil lamp. Take a moment to honour and remember the soul who is no longer here in physical form. You may wish to silently repeat these words:

In my heart, I hold the light of your soul.
I honour your soul so pure and bright.
May love and peace bless us both. In my
heart, I forever hold the light of your soul.

Spend a few moments in silence before bringing the ceremony to a close when you are ready. Allow the candle to completely extinguish on its own if it is safe to do so. You can keep the flower or release it in a nearby stream or river or the sea.

⏸ *Healing after loss blessing ceremony*

For this ceremony you will need:

- 1 cup myrrh resin (myrrh balances emotions and promotes grounding)
- 1 cup palo santo chips (palo santo supports healing)
- 1 cup frankincense resin (frankincense promotes calm and peace)
- 6 drops rose essential oil (rose has high vibration properties, opens the heart chakra and invites love)
- special items of your choice such as shells, crystals or a photo
- a small tray
- white roses
- incense tongs
- a charcoal tablet
- a stone bowl filled with sand
- a white candle or a tea light

Be clear about your intention before you start the ceremony. Repeat silently:

> *I am here to heal. I am ready to receive healing and guidance on my healing journey.*

Grind the myrrh, palo santo chips and frankincense then add the essential oil and mix well. While you are grinding and mixing the ingredients, thank them for their healing properties. If you would like to make enough just for one ceremony, adjust the quantities; for example, 1 teaspoon of dry ingredients and one drop of rose essential oil. You can also buy a ready-made incense blend. Store the incense mix in an airtight jar that has been labelled.

Place some items that hold special meaning for you on the tray and add some white flowers (white symbolises purity, peace and innocence as well as new beginnings). When you are ready to begin, sit or stand and place the tray in front of you. Take a few cleansing breaths to clear your mind and bring your attention to the here and now. Make your intention clear; meet yourself where you are right at this moment.

Hold the charcoal tablet with incense tongs and light the other end before placing it in the stone bowl.

Sprinkle the incense blend on the hot charcoal and light the white candle (white especially represents light in its highest spiritual frequency and embraces female mysteries; it is both the protector and the giver). As you light the candle invite only pure healing energy into your space, and as you breathe in acknowledge all the raw, tangled up, fuzzy emotions that have visited you since your loss. Acknowledge just one emotion at a time and take your time. As you exhale, allow each emotion to flow away from you.

Visualise, sense and feel the emotions being cleansed by the smoke of the incense and being replaced by pure healing energy, light and love. Silently repeat this prayer:

I tend to my broken heart with love and kindness. Let love and peace flow to the deepest, emptiest and darkest corners of my being. I am ready to receive healing and guidance from the universe. I am healing each and every day.

You can replace the word 'universe' with another word that resonates with you; for example, God, spirit, angels or source.

Every time you breath in, fill your heart with gratitude. Every time you breathe out, send love and gratitude to everyone who has been part of this journey with you.

When you are ready, slowly open your eyes. Take a moment to return to your present surrounding, and end the ceremony with a grateful heart for having been blessed by having had the deceased in your life and for having known the deceased even if it was for a very brief moment.

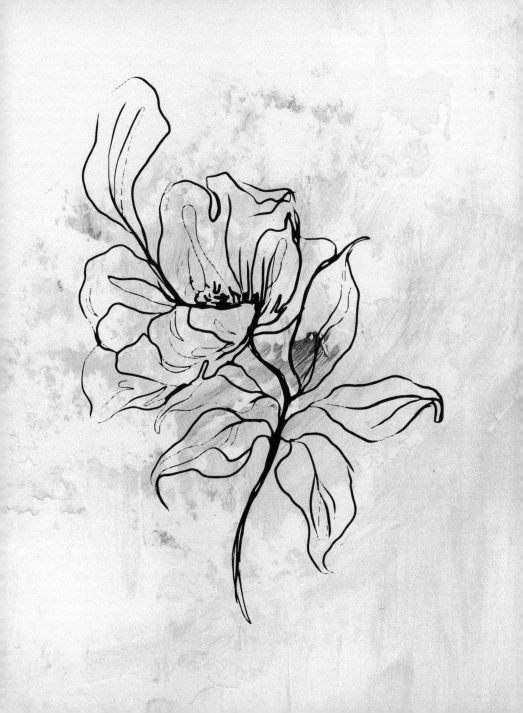

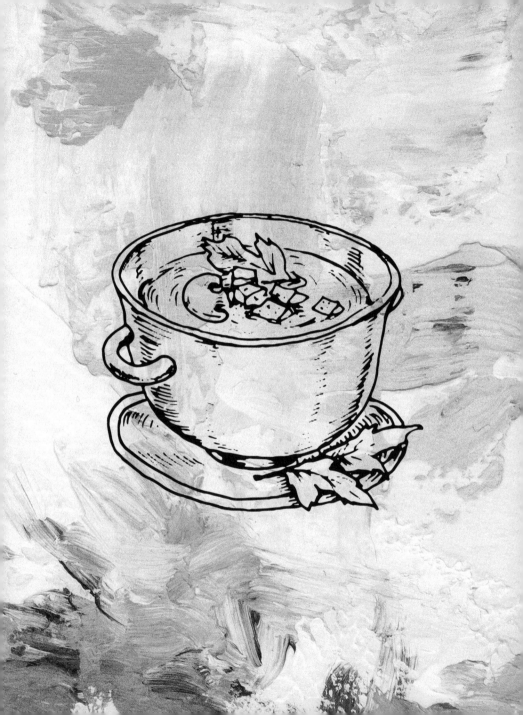

20

Foods that will promote healing

revitalise from within

Healing is as much physical as it is emotional, so in this chapter the attention is moved to the body. Nutritious food will heal your cells from the inside and help you to find balance, and a strong body will make it easier for you to take care of your emotions as you continue your journey through grief.

Grief can adversely affect your appetite: you may not want to eat, and when you do you may turn to fast and processed foods. We all have different relationships with food, and in times of sorrow we may adopt unhealthy eating habits.

We have all heard the saying 'treat your body as a temple', so this chapter focuses on restoring your physical health with healing foods. Herbal infusions and recipes that will give your body a boost and maintain your physical health have been included.

● *Kitchen ritual*

The kitchen is the heart of your home. Give your kitchen a good clean and clear the cupboards of expired and unhealthy processed foods. Transform your kitchen into a recovery hub in which you can create healing infusions and meals; a clean, uncluttered work surface will help you set your intention when you are preparing your meals.

It is always good practice to give thanks to the vegetables, plants and ingredients you use in your cooking. With every stir of the pot, infuse the food with loving and healing energy and with joy. Before you take a sip of your herbal infusion or meal, you may want to close your eyes, bring your attention to the food in front of you and silently repeat this small blessing:

I am grateful for the food I am about to eat.
May this food help heal and nourish my body.

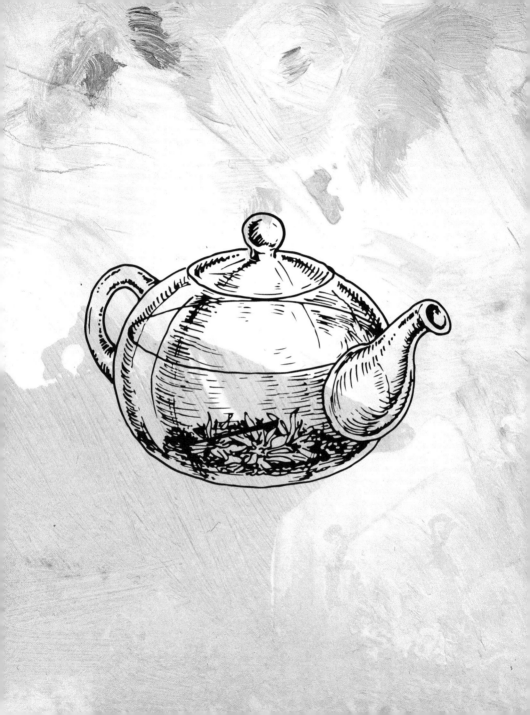

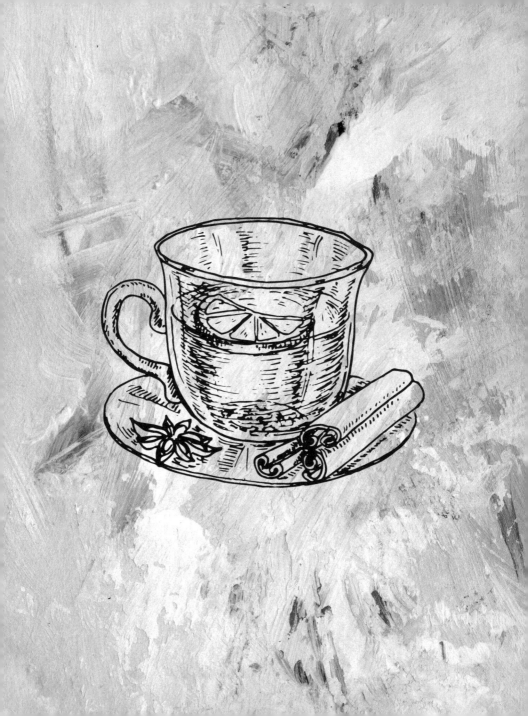

Herbal infusions recipes

Herbal infusions or teas are a simple and inexpensive means to harvest the healing, soothing and restorative properties of herbs. When making herbal infusions, it is best to use filtered water to retain the flavour of the herbs. Below is a handful of recipes that were especially chosen for their rich, healing benefits. They are particularly good for restoring and maintaining your digestive health as well as your overall physical health. Some are based on traditional Chinese medicine and others are recipes that were adapted from my native island of Mauritius.

● *Goji berry herbal infusion*

I start with goji berries as it is probably the easiest herbal infusion recipe. Goji berries, also known as wolfberries, are considered to be a herb tonic in Chinese medicine. Choose good-quality dried berries, which are easy to spot as they tend to be a nice reddish colour and slightly more puffy.

Method:

1. Rinse 1 tablespoon of dried goji berries with water, then place them in a teapot and pour over 2 cups of hot water. Cover and let it steep for about one hour. Strain the tea into a cup and snack on the hydrated berries while you drink the tea.

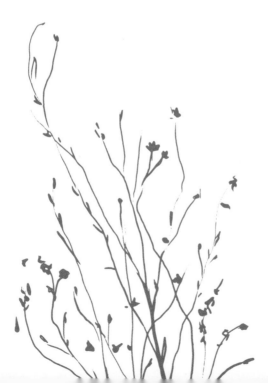

THE ART OF GRIEVING

ⅠⅠ *Turmeric herbal infusion*

When turmeric is used wisely it can restore balance in your body, help with reducing menstruation pain, improving blood and energy flow, and can boost digestion. Turmeric has anti-inflammatory properties that make it a good ally in preventing certain illnesses. Avoid turmeric if you are on any blood-thinning medication, are pregnant or are anaemic. It is also best to avoid it if you feel very weak and have a very pale complexion.

For this delicious warming tea you will need:

- 500 ml rice milk
- 5 cm piece fresh turmeric peeled and crushed into a paste (or substitute with 1 teaspoon ground turmeric)
- 6 –7 green cardamom pods lightly crushed to open the pods
- 1 cinnamon stick
- 3 whole cloves
- pinch black pepper
- muscovado or dark brown sugar, to taste

Method:

1. Place the first six ingredients into a pot and bring the mixture gently to the boil, reducing the heat as soon as it starts to boil. Simmer gently for 10 minutes. Strain into a cup and add the sugar.

⦿ *Spearmint infusion*

Spearmint is a cooling herb that is great for digestion and for its ability to help balance emotions and reduce anxiety. Good digestion and balanced emotions are important, because the heart and small intestine make a yin/yang pair, and when inflammation blockages are removed from the digestive tract the heart becomes calmer. You will be less prone to being irritable or quick to anger. When combined with fennel seeds, spearmint can reduce abdominal bloating after meals.

To make a spearmint infusion blend you will need:

- 4 tablespoons fennel seeds
- ½ teaspoon black peppercorns
- 1 cup dried spearmint leaves

Method:

1. Gently crush the fennel seeds and peppercorns then mix in the spearmint and stir to combine. Store in an airtight jar.

2. To enjoy this infusion, add a teaspoon or two of the blend to a small teapot, pour over hot water and let it steep for five minutes before straining into a cup.

ⅣV *Ginger elixir*

An aromatic herb used in Asian cuisine, ginger is a warming condiment that is excellent for giving your immune system a boost.

To make this elixir you will need:

- 8 cm piece fresh ginger, peeled
- 1 litre filtered water
- muscovado sugar or good-quality organic honey, to taste

Method:

1. Place the ginger and water in a blender and give it a good whizz. Pour into a saucepan and bring gently to the boil. Allow to simmer over a low heat for about 10 minutes with the lid on. To serve, strain into a cup and add the sugar or honey. In warmer weather you may like to enjoy this delicious elixir cool, in which case add half a cup to some freshly squeezed orange juice and sweeten with the sugar.

2. You can strain the remaining mixture into a preserving jar or bottle and store it in the fridge, then easily reheat enough for a cup whenever you fancy a warming tea. This mixture will keep for a couple of weeks.

Ⓥ *Nettle and cardamom infusion*

Nettle is considered to be a tonic herb and can be beneficial if you have poor appetite. Cardamom is well known as a warming herb and is excellent for the stomach and digestion.

To make one large cup of nettle tea, you will need:

- 3–4 green cardamom pods
- 250 ml water
- 1 teaspoon dried nettle
- raw honey or muscovado sugar, to taste

Method:

1. Slightly crush the cardamom pods just enough to open them. Bring the water gently to the boil, then reduce the heat and add the nettle and cardamom pods to the pan. Cover and simmer for five minutes before turning the heat off. Allow the infusion to steep until cool enough to drink and strain into a cup. Add a little honey or sugar.

Ⓥ *Green chai infusion*

I use gunpowder green tea for this infusion, which is perfect if you need a boost in the morning or if you have difficulty making the transition from summer to autumn. As green tea contains caffeine you should avoid it if you are on medication for heart problems, depression or anxiety as it may interfere with the absorption of the medication. The recipe below is for a batch that is large enough to share or store in the fridge and use the next day.

For this infusion you will need:

- 500 ml filtered water
- 250 ml rice milk
- 1 tablespoon gunpowder green tea
- ½ teaspoon fresh crushed ginger
- ¼ teaspoon black peppercorns, crushed
- 8 green cardamom pods
- 1 star anise
- 1 cinnamon stick
- muscovado sugar, to taste

Method:

1. Pour the water and rice milk into a saucepan and bring gently to the boil, then reduce the heat before adding all of the remaining ingredients except the sugar. Simmer over a very low heat for a further 10 minutes, then strain into a cup and add the sugar.

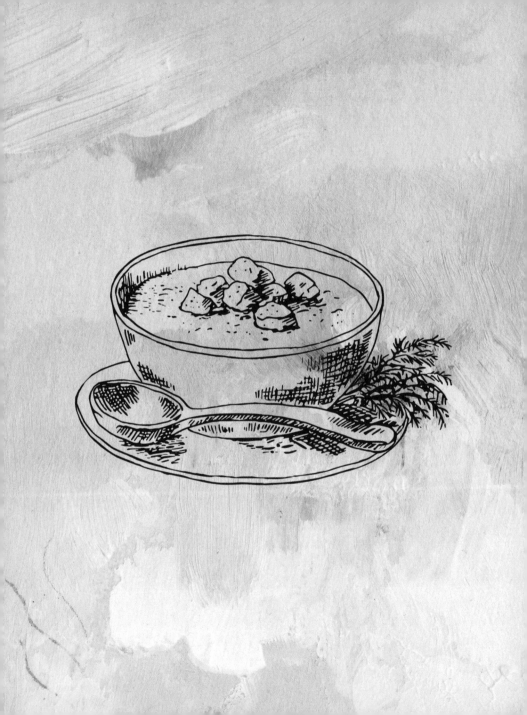

Comforting soups

One of my childhood memories is of my mother giving me a bowl of chicken soup whenever I had a cold. Perhaps it was the love the soup had been prepared with rather than the chicken soup itself that helped; perhaps it was both! Soup became my favourite dish every time I needed a pick me up on cold, dreary days. Soups and meals prepared with great care, intention and love become healers of body and soul and are so easy to make. I have included some of my favourite go-to soup recipes, which are nourishing and comforting although they are spicy, so if you do not tolerate spices very well use half the amount listed. As you prepare the soup, set your intention. Thank the ingredients for their healing properties and sprinkle the soup with love.

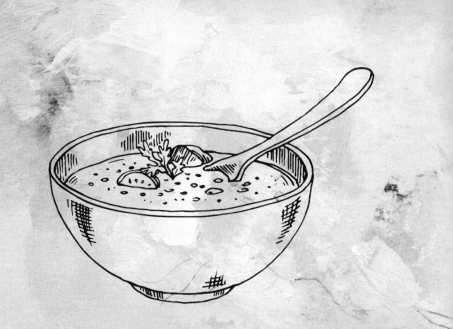

① *Spicy carrot and coriander coconut soup*

Carrots are often recommended in traditional Chinese medicine to tonify the qi (energy) and to strengthen all the organs. Inexpensive, full of minerals, rich in various nutrients and often found in abundance in markets, carrots are the perfect vegetables; you can cook them in many different ways and even juice them. This warming soup would be ideal for lunch or dinner.

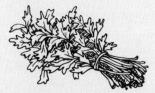

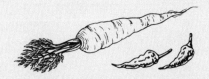

You will need:

- 1 tablespoon coriander seeds
- 1 tablespoon coconut or grapeseed oil
- 4 garlic cloves, finely chopped
- ½ teaspoon fresh ginger, finely chopped
- 1 small shallot, finely chopped
- 1 tablespoon mild curry powder
- ¼ teaspoon of dried chilli flakes
- 450 g organic carrots, peeled and chopped
- 300 ml unsweetened coconut milk
- 1 litre vegetable stock
- 1 big bunch fresh coriander
- salt and pepper, to taste

Method:

1. Crush the coriander seeds in a mortar and pestle to release their flavour. Gently heat the oil in a heavy-bottomed pot then add the garlic, ginger and shallot. Once the garlic and shallot have softened, add the crushed coriander seeds, curry powder, chilli flakes and carrots. Stir well for a couple of minutes before adding the coconut milk and stock and cook until the carrots are soft.

2. Finely chop two-thirds of the fresh coriander, including the stalks, add to the pot and reduce the heat. Cook while stirring for a few minutes and add the salt and pepper. Allow the soup to cool before puréeing in a blender until smooth. Gently reheat before serving.

3. You can top the soup with a crunchy carrot salad made just before you are ready to serve. Combine two peeled and grated carrots, 2 tablespoons of finely chopped spring onions and coriander leaves and add 1 tablespoon of pumpkin seeds if you like a bit of crunchiness. Season and top with the fresh carrot salad before serving with warm bread.

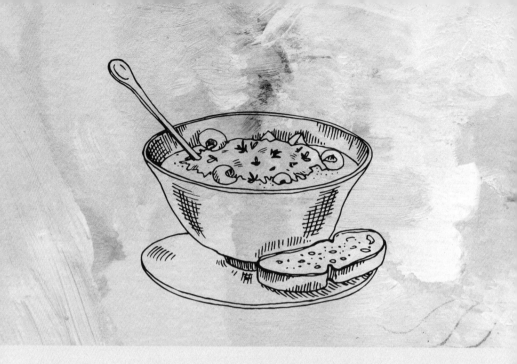

🍴 *Masoor dal (Indian red lentil soup) with spinach*

Dal is easy and quick to prepare. Packed full of protein, iron, magnesium, folate and other nutrients, it is a must to have in your kitchen pantry. If you like spices and flavours from India this soup will soon become a favourite; a bowl is guaranteed to bring comfort after a long day or on a cold, rainy evening. The soup can be served with naan bread, chapatti or white or brown rice.

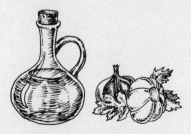

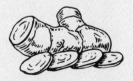

You will need:

- 200 g red lentils
- 1 tablespoon ghee or grapeseed oil
- 1 teaspoon fresh garlic, crushed
- ½ teaspoon fresh ginger, crushed
- 1 teaspoon ground coriander
- 1 teaspoon ground cumin
- ½ teaspoon garam masala
- 1 teaspoon mehti (fenugreek)
- ¼ teaspoon chilli powder
- ½ teaspoon ground turmeric
- 1 litre vegetable stock
- 2 generous handfuls fresh spinach, washed
- salt and pepper, to taste
- 1 tablespoon fresh coriander leaves, chopped

Method:

1. Wash the lentils until the water runs clear, then place in a bowl with fresh water and allow to soak for a good eight hours or overnight.

2. Put the ghee or grapeseed oil, garlic and ginger into a pan and stir well over a medium heat. Reduce the heat if the garlic and ginger start to burn. Once the garlic and ginger have softened, add the ground coriander, ground cumin, garam masala, fenugreek, chilli powder, and ground turmeric. Stir well, adding a tablespoon of water if the paste is too thick.

3. Drain the lentils then rinse once more under running water before adding them to the pan together with the vegetable stock. Cook over a medium heat until the lentils are soft then add the spinach and salt and pepper. Before serving, sprinkle over the fresh coriander.

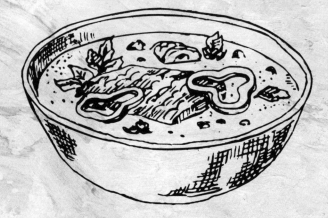

⬤ *Roasted zucchini and capsicum soup*

Zucchini and capsicum are an excellent combination that will aid digestion. While the vegetables are roasting in the oven you can enjoy a warm cup of tea, read a book or doodle in your journal. This delicious soup is easy to throw together and has the perfect yin and yang balance with its warming and cooling properties.

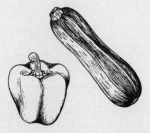

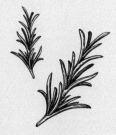

You will need:

- 2 red capsicums, roughly chopped
- 3 zucchini, roughly chopped
- 2½ tablespoons grapeseed oil
- 4 garlic cloves, finely chopped
- 1 onion, roughly chopped
- ½ teaspoon dried rosemary
- ½ teaspoon dried thyme
- ½ teaspoon dried oregano
- ½ teaspoon of dried marjoram
- 1 litre vegetable stock
- 150 g grated Parmesan cheese plus extra to serve
- salt and pepper, to taste

Method:

1. Pre-heat the oven to 185°C.

2. Put the capsicums and zucchini in a large bowl and coat them well with the oil, then add the garlic, onion and dried herbs. Mix well. Transfer to a baking tray and roast in the oven for at least 40 minutes.

3. Once the vegetables are nicely roasted, remove the tray from the oven. Heat the stock in a large pot then add the vegetables. Stir well and simmer for about 15 minutes.

4. Remove from the stove and cool before puréeing until smooth. Return to the stove to warm up and add the Parmesan cheese and salt and pepper. To serve, top with the extra grated Parmesan.

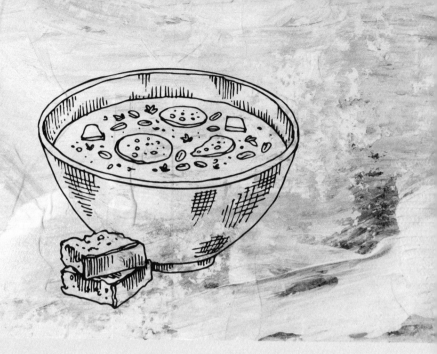

IV *Leek and potato soup*

In this humble bowl of soup you'll find the following healing gems: warmth, abundant nutrients and the ability to improve appetite and digestion. It is so creamy, comforting, delicious and easy to make it will soon become a winter staple for you and your loved ones. As an additional bonus, it freezes well when you have leftovers. Leeks and potatoes are a great combination in terms of their mild flavour and nutrition. If you find the flavour too mild, you can easily spice up the soup with a generous amount of black pepper. The fragrance of the herbs adds a comforting and delicate touch to the leeks and potatoes.

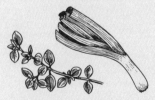

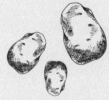

THE ART OF GRIEVING

You will need:

- 4 large leeks
- 3 medium potatoes
- 1 tablespoon grapeseed oil
- 25 g butter
- 2 garlic cloves, finely chopped
- 1 onion, finely chopped
- ¼ teaspoon dried tarragon
- 1 teaspoon thyme
- 1.2 litres vegetable stock, heated
- 200 ml crème fraiche
- salt and black pepper, to taste

Method:

1. Chop the leeks, using only the white and light green parts. Rinse well and set aside. Peel the potatoes and cut into small cubes. Gently heat the oil and butter in a heavy-bottomed pan, then add the garlic and onion. Once the onion and garlic have softened, toss in the potatoes and stir well before adding the leeks. Give it another good stir.

2. Add the dried tarragon and thyme and pour in the hot vegetable stock. Increase the heat and cook until the leek and potatoes are soft. Turn off the heat and puree with a hand-held blender until smooth. If you are using a conventional blender, allow the soup to cool first.

3. Pour the soup into a clean pot and return to the stove over a gentle heat. Stir in the crème fraiche and salt and pepper. Have extra black pepper to season when you are ready to serve.

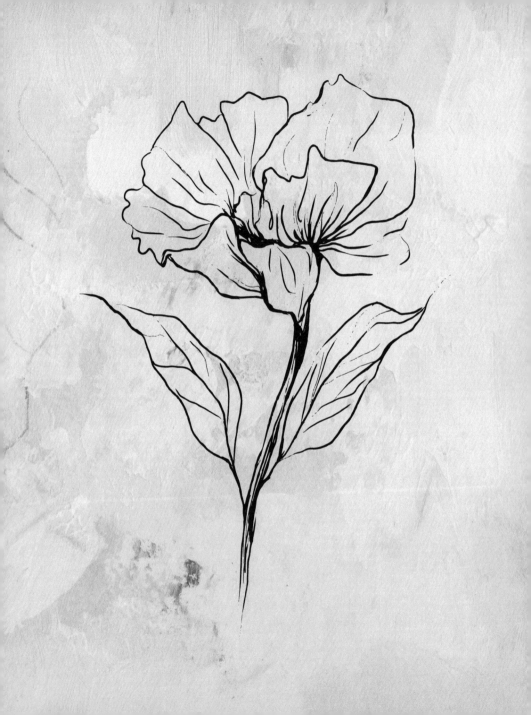

A final word

Do not fear grief, for it is a natural process and a partner in your healing.

I hope this book has helped you discover your ability to heal. I hope it has helped you uncover the hidden resources you already possess. I hope that through engaging with the self-care rituals and creative activities shared in this book the dark, heavy clouds of grief have lifted enough to allow you to tap into the divine spark of living a fulfilled, joyful life that is free of guilt.

Remember: your healing is an ongoing process so always be gentle and compassionate with yourself. Always return to love.

Here are some lines from one of my favourite poets, Rabindranath Tagore:

When I stand before thee at the day's end,
thou shalt see my scars and know that I
had my wounds and also my healing.

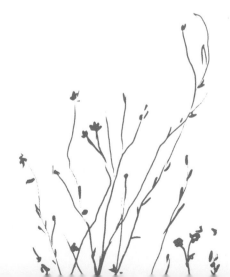

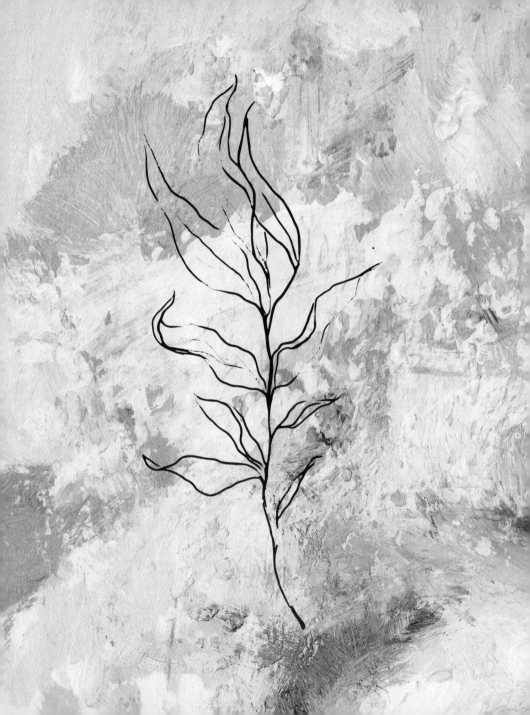

Bibliography

Chia, Mantak and William U. Wei, 2013, *Chi Nei Ching: Muscle, tendon and meridian massage*, Destiny Books, Vermont

Gilbert, Elizabeth, 2016, *Big Magic: Creative living beyond fear*, Riverhead Books, New York

Kinkele, Thomas, 2004, *Incense and Incense Rituals: Healing ceremonies for spaces of subtle energy*, Lotus Press, USA

Kumar, Sameet M., 2013, *Mindfulness for Prolonged Grief: A guide to healing after loss when depression, anxiety and anger won't go away*, New Harbinger Publications, USA

Permutt, Philip, 2016, *The Crystal Healer: Crystal prescriptions that will change your life forever*, CICO Books, USA

Quinlan, Ginger, 2012, *Scents of the Soul: Creating herbal incense for mind, body and soul*, Findhorn Press, Scotland

Thich Nhat Hanh, 1990, *Transformation & Healing: the Sutra on the four establishments of mindfulness*, Parallax Press, California

Wagyal Rinpoche, Tenzin, 2015, *The True Source of Healing: How the ancient Tibetan practice of soul retrieval can transform and enrich your life*, Hay House, USA

Worwood, Valerie Ann, 2006, *Aromatherapy for the Soul: Healing the spirit with fragrance and essential oils*, New World Library, USA

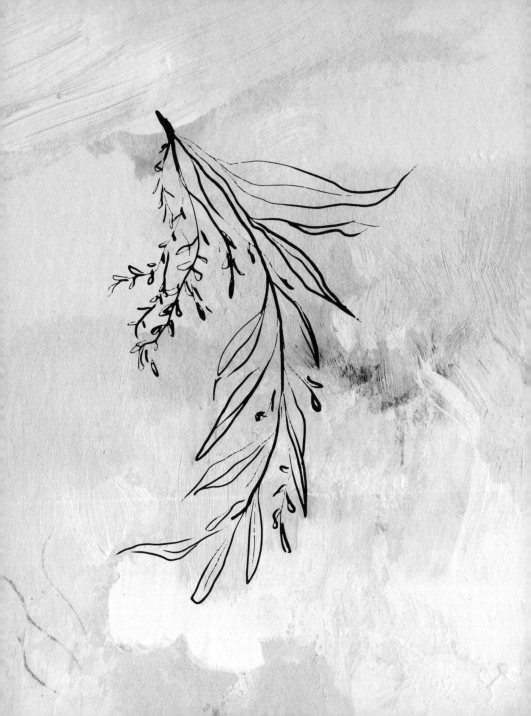

About the author

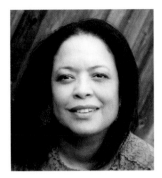

Corinne Laan, a licensed acupuncturist and traditional Chinese medicine (TCM) practitioner, runs an acupuncture practice in Amsterdam that specialises in women's health.

As a former specialist nurse and natural healer Corinne became fascinated by the human psyche and the mind/body connection. This, coupled with her own personal quest and desire for self-healing, sent her on a journey of self-development. An encounter with a spiritual coach encouraged her to claim her true calling and become a beacon of hope for those navigating the hardest and darkest chapter in their lives.

Corinne dived deeper into various healing methods from her heritage and adopted other practices she came across on her path. While studying TCM she encountered *yang sheng*: the philosophy of nourishing life. The concept of optimising health and well-being through nurturing mind, body and spirit became her new passion, a passion she shares with her clients.

Corinne weaves her intuition, wisdom, compassion and empathy into her work.

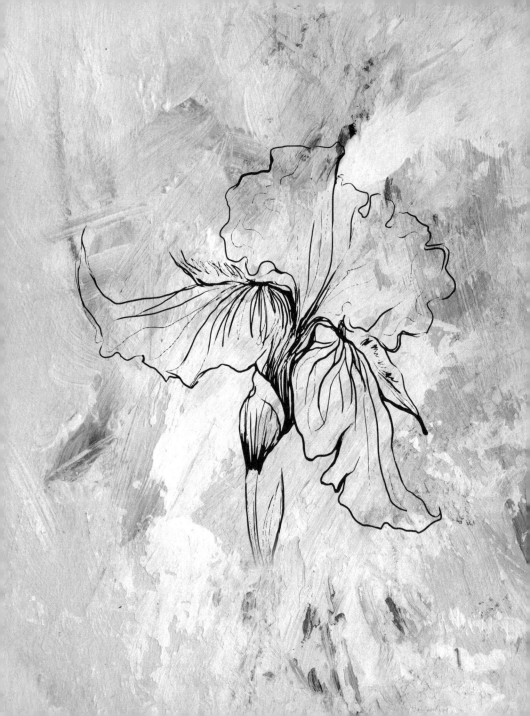

As you step into

a new tomorrow

may you remember

you are the master

of your own grief.